Our Love Multiplied

One decision. Two families.
A mother's unforgettable true story.

*For Becky Monroe—
I never met you, yet I miss you deeply.
Your life blessed mine, and I look forward to the day that
heaven brings us together.*

Copyright © 2025 Brooke Martin.

All rights reserved.

No part of this book may be reproduced, distributed, or transmitted in any form or by any means, whether electronic or mechanical, including photocopying, recording, inclusion in AI systems, or by any information storage and retrieval system, without permission in writing from the author.

Cover design: Brooke Martin.
Interior design and ebook conversion: Tod McCoy.

ISBN: 9798275649215 (softcover)
ISBN: 9798276785912 (hardcover)

Table of Contents

Forward   7

Part 1—The Martins   9
The order of things   9
Facing infertility   14
Living our lives   16
Faith and IVF   21
Twins   25
Me? Pregnant?   26
No sleep and an embryo decision   31
Being a stay-at-home mom   34
Not again!   38
Busy days in Colorado   40
Twin talents and hobbies   44

Part 2—The Connection   55
The call   55
Telling our boys   75
Getting to know each other   77

Part 3—The Monroes   91
The Monroes' journey   92
Fear   99
Three of everything   101
More miracles   103
A community of support   104
Triplet toddler years   105
So many similarities!   106
Learning about their biological origin   107
The diagnosis   108
DNA search   109

Part 4—The Meeting   117
The first meeting   117
Family reunion   126
Going viral   127

Part 5—Full Circle   143

Epilogue   149

Forward

As Brooke Martin's husband, I want you to know that every word in this book is the result of decades of deep love, countless prayers, and thoughtful reflection. What you're about to read comes straight from her heart.

Brooke has been faithful for as long as I've known her—faithful to God, to our family, and to the journey we've walked together. Like many of us, she's wrestled with impatience at times, wondering how our story would unfold, questioning the timing and plan. But through it all, her trust in God never wavered for long. She is a devoted mother and a loving wife, and her strength has been a foundation in our home.

Life, of course, throws its share of curveballs. But together, we've leaned on our faith—believing wholeheartedly that with God, all things are possible. When challenges came, we caught them and tossed them back with the same determination and hope that has guided us since day one.

This story—our story—has only taken shape because Brooke has continually sought God's voice and His guidance. She still does, every single day.

So, as you turn the pages of this book and walk through the journey it tells, know that it's not just Brooke's story—it's ours. A family story. One built on faith, love, and the incredible grace of God.

With all my love,

Chris

Part 1—The Martins

The order of things

There's a famous episode of the TV show *Friends* that depicts the group trying to hoist a couch up a flight of stairs. After planning how to get it done, the group tries to lift the long, straight couch up the 90-degree angle of the stairs, and it doesn't fit. So the character Ross yells: "PIVOT!" But pivoting a couch is difficult in a tight space, and eventually the bulky furniture got stuck. Like that couch, life can present curveballs which leave us scrambling and trying to navigate a space that feels impossibly tight. People can get stuck.

We plan so carefully and when changes hit, we try our best to "pivot." I have to admit that the majority of my own pivots have been in reaction to things I couldn't control.

In my early 20s, my parents got divorced after being married for 27 years. It was a complete shock, and having been married only a few years myself, I remember that seismic shift which changed my view of marriage. I was hit with the realization that marriage wasn't always going to be rosy like I thought it would be. As far as I knew, my parents never fought and had few disagreements. I thought that's the way it was supposed to be. I learned early in my life to avoid conflict by being very agreeable and positive. Being argumentative was not in my DNA, so when I married into a family that was loud and not afraid of confrontation, it was a shock. I had to adjust my expectations and learn that love within a family is shown in many different ways.

Another event that changed me was the death of my father in 1994. He was an extremely intelligent man and was a music professor most of his life. A high-achieving Fulbright Scholar, he played French Horn and was chosen to study in Austria in his twenties. Although he was a musician, he had the mind of a businessman.

He was always looking for the fast-money scheme. After leaving his teaching job of over 20 years, he held several sales jobs that did not go well, working late nights selling windows in people's homes, then working for a company that made folding cardboard boxes of different sizes that were used by retail industries. Due to many of his life disappointments, including the divorce from my mother, my father plummeted into a deep depression and never recovered. He quit caring about himself and for his health. He was a chain smoker and loved his bourbon, and he refused to go to the doctor or take medication for his high blood pressure. When he died in his sleep at the young age of fifty-six, it was a shock. He got stuck.

Now that I'm getting older—knocking 60—I realize that things are knit together in our lives in a certain order for a certain reason. When I was in my 20s and 30s, it was difficult if not impossible to see that. I thought I was so wise. But it turns out that I was "building my testimony" in my younger years. I was living through hard times in life which would build up my emotional, physical, and spiritual strength to use later in life.

Getting married, having a career, having a family—all of that seems so random at times. Life events did not happen in the way that I thought they would, but reflecting now, I see that God had His hand in the order of events. Many directions of life are presented to us, and it's up to us to choose which path to take. Sure, I had choices, and I made some bad ones along the way, but He used those to direct my path so that I am exactly where I am today. The bad choices taught me to appreciate the difficulty and payoff of the good choices.

Another pivot was waiting 12 years after getting married to have children. That wait was caused by infertility problems.

I can't say that I was ever one of those women who had a burning desire to have babies. My mom was an artist, an art professor, and a career woman. Growing up on the campus of Tennessee Technological University in Cookeville, Tennessee, exposed me to the fact that women could be professionals, teachers, and much more than a 50s-version of a housewife. I didn't know many stay-at-home moms when I was growing up; most of my mother's friends were teachers or had some sort of career.

    I was a 1970's latchkey kid. I came home from school to watch Gilligan's Island and The Brady Bunch while doing homework, then sometimes even started supper for the family before my parents got home. It was a good childhood with lots of freedom—riding bikes around the neighborhood with my best friend Joanna and going to the skating rink on the weekends. I took piano lessons and dance lessons, and I was in many summer musicals and dance performances. I was the "good girl" growing up. As far as I can remember, I never got in trouble or was disrespectful to my parents. I was a rule-follower and graduated seventh in my high school class of three hundred-fifty students.

    Growing up, I was outgoing with the positive attitude I inherited from my mother. I was always a "glass is always more than half full" person.

    I was also obsessed with news stories and have vivid memories of getting up at 4AM to watch the wedding of Princess Diana in 1981. The excitement of viewing breaking news and true-to-life stories of celebrities piqued my interest so much that I decided I wanted to be a news anchor when I grew up. Motherhood was not put at the forefront of my goals, but I did always want to be a wife.

    After having a few boyfriends in high school and early college, I met auburn-headed Chris Martin in August of 1986, while I was starting my junior year of college at Tennessee Tech. I majored in Journalism and got my license to be a radio announcer as part of the educational program. I got a job at a local pop radio station called Jet 107 as the "news girl." Chris was the night DJ. He was originally from Sparta, Tennessee, and had started working in the radio industry when he was asked to give play-by-plays of local football games at WSMT radio station in Sparta. He also had gotten his radio license and had worked there for a few years.

    Chris always wore a denim jacket and was a bit of a "bad boy." I thought he was cute, but apparently he thought I was a stuck-up sorority girl. My mom was a faculty advisor for the ADPi sorority on campus, so I joined the sorority when I was a freshman. Because I was living in the same town I grew up in, I didn't feel a huge need to make new friends. I was involved in the sorority but not to the extent that others were. Overall, I didn't date "fraternity guys", and when Chris and I met at the radio station, I was dating someone else who was not in a fraternity. When I broke up with my boyfriend, I went to a local nightclub, the Amvets Post 40, to have some fun. Turns out, Chris was the DJ at the nightclub, and we recognized each other from Jet 107. After that first dance—probably to an 80's hair band—we started dating. Truth be told, I was the one that followed up with a phone call to him.

Chris' personality was, and is still, of a confident, decisive man. To say he is very sure of himself is an understatement, and that is what drew me to him. He had already sown some wild oats, and he had even taken a break from college and moved to Fort Worth, Texas, for a year before moving back and continuing his education. Ironically, at the time we met, my parents had moved temporarily to Fort Worth, where my mother was getting her Master's Degree in Art from Texas Christian University. I lived with two roommates in a small apartment off campus in Cookeville. My mother always wondered if the reason I got together with Chris was because they moved away. Chris provided solid decision-making that made me feel safe and protected.

Although we knew we wanted to eventually get married, the plan was for Chris to meet my parents, who were still living in Fort Worth, before we got engaged. But Chris proposed only four months after we met, on December 21st, 1986. The engagement fell on the shortest day of the year, the first day of winter, which is easy to remember. When we flew to Fort Worth for Christmas, I showed up with a marquis-shaped diamond cluster on my hand.

While visiting my parents, it was decided that we would go ahead and get married that summer, on July 25, 1987. It was seven months of whirlwind wedding planning!

The wedding day was one of the hottest days of the year in Cookeville, and we were married in a fully choreographed ceremony at the Cookeville First United Presbyterian Church. The music was perfect, and my dress was a white 1980's puff-sleeved with a long train. My bridesmaids were in shiny mauve handmade dresses with rose-shaped shoulders, and the flowers and boutonnieres matched the bridesmaid colors. More than 400 people attended our wedding; it was the event of the summer in our small town. We rode from the church to the reception in an antique Thunderbird convertible that belonged to one of the richest families in town. I was 20 and Chris was twenty-two.

We moved into married student housing on campus, which were white, cinder block apartments with barely enough room to turn around in the kitchen. I continued to go to school and finish my degree in journalism, but Chris needed to complete student teaching for his degree in health and physical education. Several of the teachers in that department were less than understanding about his need to keep his job and were inflexible on timing of tests. So we decided that he would get a full-time job and work hard while I finished my degree and worked part-time. I graduated in August of 1988 with my Bachelor of Science degree in journalism and got a job as a reporter at the Sparta Expositor in Sparta, Tennessee. By this time, Chris had worked his way up in the restaurant industry and was the manager of the Sparta Pizza Hut.

Over the next few years, we worked hard and built our dream house in Sparta, with three acres on the Calfkiller River. Our home included three bedrooms, 2 ½ baths, with a hot tub on our back deck surrounded by trees. The sprawling house had a huge room above what would have been a garage if it would have been a one-level house. We turned that room into a TV room with a huge bar that we bought from a fraternity house at Tennessee Tech.

We enjoyed our time with friends and family there and spent many weekends hosting parties. Chris became known as "The Pizza Man," and after following ambulances to the White County Hospital as a news reporter, I was offered a job as the marketing director there. I enjoyed the position, managing hospital events, school tours and the hospital's senior volunteer program. Chris also had a fancy fish/ski boat that we would take out on Center Hill Lake many weekends. Between work and fun, we honestly were not thinking about starting a family yet.

But like many couples, by our late 20's we decided it was

time to try to have children. Both sets of potential grandparents were asking for grandchildren, and we didn't want to wait much longer. However, after about a year with no success, we realized we needed to see if there was anything wrong with either one of our reproductive systems. The infertility industry was still fairly young at that time. We started the process by going to Dr. Harry Stuber, the OB/GYN in Cookeville who I had been going to for years, who also did infertility testing. I was 28 years old.

Facing infertility

The testing over the next several months made me feel like a science experiment. My menstrual cycles were regular, and there was nothing indicating any other obvious problems. The first step was having a hysterosalpingogram—a procedure which involves shooting dye into my fallopian tubes and watching on x-ray to see whether they are open and able to transport the egg to the uterus to be fertilized and implanted. I recalled that, over the years, I had experienced some shooting-type pains in my abdomen, almost like having a "stitch" in my lower stomach. I always wondered if that had something to do with infertility problems. The test immediately revealed the issue: both of my tubes were completely closed for unknown reasons—possibly infection in the past. The solution was surgery to re-open the tubes and create a pathway for the eggs to travel, fertilization to happen, and implantation of the embryo to be successful. I thought the solution seemed fairly simple and made sense.

I was put to sleep with anesthesia, and the endoscopic procedure was done without having to make a big incision. There were three small puncture holes made that were able to fit the equipment and a camera. Dr. Stuber re-opened the end of the fallopian tubes into flower-shaped petals and made sure the tubes would carry fluid. Air was also pumped into the area to inflate a space for Dr. Stuber to do his work. The dissipation of the air after the procedure caused some pain in my neck and arms, but it was deemed a success. After a brief recovery, we were given the "go" to start trying again.

Within a few months, success! With a positive pregnancy test and hopes high, we started telling a few family members. But on Valentine's Day, 1995, when I was about four weeks pregnant, I was on my way to a work appointment, driving my car on bumpy country roads. I started having severe pain in my right lower abdomen and quickly called my husband, then the doctor.

I was rushed into Dr. Stuber's office to get an ultrasound, which discovered an ectopic pregnancy. The egg had traveled up the fallopian tube, been fertilized, and the embryo had gotten stuck in the fallopian tube, which still apparently had some damage from years of being closed and filled with fluid. I had heard that tubal pregnancies could be life-threatening due to the internal bleeding they can cause. It was a scary situation, and I was glad it was diagnosed quickly. I immediately went to the hospital and had emergency surgery. It was a whirlwind, and I let Chris handle many of the details since I was in pain.

I have always been a pragmatic person and positive to a fault. I had only known for about a week that I was pregnant, so the fact that I was losing a baby never really occurred to me. I think that my friends and family were more upset than I was, but I learned a lot about my ability to pivot.

Dr. Stuber was very thorough and took the time to consult with a fertility specialist, Dr. George Hill, at the Nashville Fertility Center. He suggested removing my fallopian tubes, otherwise risk another dangerous ectopic pregnancy.

Due to the ectopic pregnancy, we learned that I could get pregnant if the egg and sperm met. But due to removal of my fallopian tubes, we would have to utilize a procedure called In Vitro Fertilization (IVF). This process would create embryos in a lab by uniting the egg and sperm in a petri dish, then the doctors would implant the successfully-fertilized embryo in my uterus. We required this method of transportation to move the embryos from the dish to my uterus.

But the whole process seemed daunting. There was no guarantee that it would work, and it was expensive; our insurance covered very little of it. Considering the cost and the unknowns at the time, we decided to wait. I was 29 at that time. We also talked about adopting a baby and were considering adopting from China. But between the cost and our lifestyle, we just weren't ready to commit to adoption or In Vitro Fertilization.

Living our lives

We had been involved in the Methodist church in town over the years. We'd been in the choir, and I even helped teach in a children's choir. Church wasn't a priority for us but more of a requirement, instilled in us through our families. However, in 1999, we encountered some bumps in our marriage. I wasn't used to conflict and thought any disagreements were the result of lacking love and understanding. Instead of becoming a part of intense or negative conversations, I tended to shut down. We went to counseling, which helped some. We worked on our communication with each other and being more transparent about our feelings and even our finances.

Some of our dear friends, Eileen and Ron Cunliffe, who had joined us in many parties, gatherings and happy hours over several years, had started going to church regularly. We both respected them so much, and they invited us to go with them. They told us about the "new hope" they had found through Jesus, and that their church was exciting.

I don't remember church ever being exciting. I was raised in a Presbyterian church which was very academic. My father was the choir director and my mother taught Sunday School, but we were never allowed to clap and act casual during the service. I was very involved in the youth group, always went to church camps and was even a delegate to a national youth conference at Purdue University in high school. I always considered myself a Christian through my actions, attending church and being involved in church activities. But, admittedly, I wasn't committed to God's plan in my life at that time.

We had heard about the church that Ron and Eileen were going to and that it was one of "those" churches where they raised their hands and clapped a lot. I remember telling Chris that if anything weird happened, we would just leave.

We decided to give Trinity Assembly in Algood, Tennessee, a try.

The first Sunday was overwhelming but, paradoxically, left me feeling tranquil. The music flowed right through me and was peaceful. There was a small choir led by Jason Yarbrough, and everyone seemed genuinely happy to be there. During the sermon, Pastor Eddie Turner walked from one end of the stage to the other in the large sanctuary filled with hundreds of people. Then he stopped in front of us and talked to us like he had been in our living room all week. He talked about life struggles that we were going through and solutions that could happen through trusting our lives and our marriage to Jesus. It was a surreal experience that took us totally by surprise.

The following week, Ron and Eileen encouraged us to attend again.

The next Sunday we went back and moved to the other side of the sanctuary, and the same thing happened. We thought it was very weird and wondered what was going on, as if a supernatural event was happening. The third Sunday, at the end of the service, Pastor Eddie did an altar call (asking if anyone wanted to come to the altar and pray the prayer of salvation). With our eyes closed, he counted to three, and when I looked up, my husband was at the altar. I froze and didn't know what to do but found myself following him then standing beside him in front of the large congregation. He was hugging Pastor Eddie and crying. It's embarrassing to say, but I was thinking, "Oh great, now we are going to try the Jesus thing!" But God soon corrected my heart and told me that I needed to follow my husband more and to follow Jesus. That life-changing day occurred on Sunday, April 18, 1999.

We had made plans after church that Sunday to have lunch with our friends Cheri and Clark Cropper. I met Cheri through work because she was the administrator of a nursing home in Sparta, and our paths also crossed through the Chamber of Commerce and healthcare-related events. Our husbands met and got along well, so we became fast friends, especially because they were near our age and, like us, had not had children yet. We knew they attended church, but surprisingly had never had many discussions about our spiritual beliefs. At lunch, as we were still processing what happened at church, we nervously told Cheri and Clark about our experience. Their response surprised me! Cheri said, "You weren't saved yet?" We spent lunch talking about salvation, God and Jesus, and our friendship continued to grow.

Within a few days, I could tell my husband was different. He was reading the Bible and seemed to gain immediate knowledge. He went from zero to 100 spiritually! On the other hand, I was slow to believe. This was a pivot I wasn't sure about. I needed proof.

Isn't it funny how God tends to not only meet those challenges we come up with—but also exceed them? I had no idea how God was going to prove himself to me, and if anyone would have told me, I would have said that they'd lost their mind. From my experiences in observing others, being a Christian was boring. No fun and no adventure. But I really did want my marriage to work, so I started seeking answers.

We attended some discipleship classes at Trinity Assembly—learning the basics of the Christian faith, and I discovered how God's Old Testament promises came true in the New Testament. I realized that historical events were foretold hundreds of years apart. I'd taken part in Bible studies as a teenager and had gone to church camp, but I never had a "relationship" with God or Jesus, and I never heard the Salvation Gospel of Jesus Christ. The need for Him to cover my sins so that I could join Him in that perfect place in Heaven was never a part of the story that I was taught—until that Sunday in April 1999. Or maybe I'd heard but didn't listen. I think many people hear that message but don't listen or aren't ready to accept it. Until that day, I didn't have an understanding that there was any other option than going to Heaven. I thought everyone did.

While not religious before, the spiritual world had always fascinated me. When I was growing up, subjects like ghosts, poltergeists, and ESP seemed like reasonable possibilities to me, since I did believe in a spiritual realm. But I thought that anything like that was against Christian beliefs. At times, my searching led me to some of the darker sides of spirituality. All of those years I never considered that God, Jesus, and The Holy Spirit were at the core of every spiritual answer. As I learned and believe now, there's a God-shaped hole in everyone's heart. We all search for things that will fill it—all types of things called spirituality—including beliefs teetering on witchcraft, idol worship, and secular replacements.

When Chris and I had the Bible—the Word of God—to stand on, it radically changed our marriage. When that God-shaped hole in our hearts was filled, a common bond came to our marriage that we had never had before.

Chris' brother Buck had become a born-again Christian several years before and had been praying for us to turn to Jesus. He gave us a Christian book about marriage called *Rocking the Roles: Building a Win-Win Marriage* by Robert Lewis and William Hendricks. That book helped rearrange our marriage in the way God designed: making the husband a servant-leader in the marriage and explained the reason a woman's role is to be obedient to her husband, in order to provide a strength that only women have. It truly "rocked our roles," and it turned me into a better wife and woman—and eventually a mom.

There were so many habits that had to change—not only in our marriage, but individually. Throughout our 20s, Chris and I had been the party hosts at our house. That huge room above our garage had the stocked bar with every type of liquor you can imagine, and nearly every weekend was a party. So, when we became Christians, we were worried about how we were going to successfully change our partying ways. We both enjoyed entertaining our friends; Chris was a gourmet cook and a skilled mixologist.

At the time, there was an older woman named Jamila Hijazi who went to our church. She was a former Muslim who had converted to Christianity. That, in itself, shocked me. One day at church, she approached us with advice. "When you come to Jesus, he accepts you as you are," she said in her thick accent. "When He wants to change something, you will know, and it won't be hard. He will change your heart." Jamila was in the choir at church, and we joined that choir the summer of 1999. They became our church family, and we spent time as a disciple of Jamila and many others.

One day during that summer of 1999, I came home from work

to find Chris sitting on our front porch, which was a bit unusual. Just sitting there, still in his Pizza Hut uniform, waiting for me. He led me to the kitchen and showed me that he had poured every bottle of liquor down the sink. The kitchen countertop was covered with empty liquor bottles. I couldn't believe it. I asked, "Even the Kahlua?" Yes, even the Kahlua.

In fact, we discovered shortly after that so much liquor was poured down the sink that it killed all of the chemicals in our septic tank, and we had to "start over" with the new chemicals. Seems funny now, but it was a cleansing for both of us, and the septic system!

And that's how it went. Jesus changed our hearts and our relationship. I learned to trust Chris more with the little things I had been picking on him about before. Previously I was very concerned about how we spent our money, where we went to eat, and details that I spent way too much time worrying about. I learned to honor him as the head of our family, and it was a good feeling.

On September 25, 1999, Chris and I renewed our wedding vows at a beautiful little church in the country called Robinson Chapel Presbyterian Church—this time with God included. Our first wedding had been a performance, and although it was beautiful, we did not include God in the same way as our wedding renewal. My mother and I handmade a simple ivory silk dress and Chris wore a suit. Pastor Eddie officiated, we shared communion, and it was attended by 10 people: our parents, and best friends Joanna and Tommy Arnhart, Cheri and Clark, and Eileen and Ron.

We were entering into a new commitment, and behind the scenes I was feeling a lot of pressure about it. I wanted to make sure that I could be the kind of wife that God wanted me to be; I even talked to Chris about it a week before the renewal ceremony. I remember very distinctly him telling me that if I wasn't 100% committed to our marriage, I needed to walk away. Looking back, I know that was an attack by the enemy, because over the next few years the Holy Spirit would be ignited in our lives. God was paving the way for huge changes, blessings and challenges in our lives. If you think being a Christian is boring, the next part of our story might change your mind.

In October of 1999, we got baptized together at Trinity Assembly. It was such a happy occasion; we both felt like we had restarted our lives. We were new people and, shortly after the baptism, we started thinking about that plan to start our family. We had been so distracted by other things that we hadn't thought seriously about "making our quiver full," as the Bible says about having babies.

"Behold, children are a heritage from the Lord, the fruit of the womb a reward. Blessed is the man whose quiver is full of them!" (Psalm 127:3 and 5)

We remembered that Dr. Stuber had consulted with Nashville Fertility Center, so we made our first appointment there to start the process for In Vitro Fertilization. The cost was a lot for us, more than $15,000 plus the cost of medicine. But we were so "high" on God, and we just KNEW that this was the plan for us.

Faith and IVF

At our first appointment, we met with Dr. Christine Whitworth and learned about the details of the IVF process. We were given a packet of information to read, which explained that the woman takes medication to shut down the female reproductive cycle—similar to menopause—then takes more medication to start it up again in a controlled environment. The medications make the ovary follicles produce multiple eggs. In a naturally conceived pregnancy, usually one (or sometimes two) eggs release into the fallopian tube once per month and travel up to the uterus where it may get fertilized and become an embryo, then attach to the uterus for a growing pregnancy. With IVF, the doctor instead retrieves eggs from the follicles before the body naturally releases them. Sometimes there are one or two eggs that are successfully retrieved and sometimes there are more. That is where our faith played a big role.

We remember the doctors presented multiple percentage rates of success based on the stage of IVF, and they were overwhelming. For instance, 70% of harvested eggs are mature enough to use,

50% of eggs will become fertilized, 50% of those will grow to the blastocyst stage and be healthy enough to transfer, 40% chance of implantation, etc. We figured, God believes in us 100% as his children, and we are going to believe 100% that this was going to be successful. That's a hard thing for other couples who have unsuccessfully gone through IVF to hear. All I can say is that we knew, without doubt, that our IVF would be successful.

The cost of IVF or any infertility treatments can be daunting. When we went through IVF in the year 2000, very few insurance companies had coverage for it. My insurance covered the doctor's visits and the lab work. We spent the last few months of 1999 planning and saving, even dipping into our 401K and using our income tax return money.

We anticipated a cost of close to $3000 for the medications alone, which was one of the first out-of-pocket costs. When I went to pick up the first injection vials of Lupron at the Kroger pharmacy, we expected upwards of three hundred dollars. The cashier said "$40 copay." I recall asking, "Are you telling me that when I walk out of here with this medication, the transaction is done, and they won't come ask for more?" The pharmacist laughed and looked at the prescription again, and she stated that since the medication was also used to treat Menopause, my insurance covered it! To say I danced out of Kroger is an understatement.

To this day, we cannot explain how we paid for our appointments and procedures. Each appointment came, and we found a way to pay for it. Each procedure came, and God provided. Our advice to anyone going through IVF: don't live in percentages, and expect miracles.

Many of the injections were very time-sensitive, and we specifically remember once stopping to administer an injection while sitting in our red Ford F150 in the Cookeville Mall parking lot, hiding the needles to make sure no one thought we were doing illegal drugs. During that same period of time, there were countless trips to the fertility clinic (1.5 hours away), multiple blood draws and ultrasounds, (and my moodiness, according to my husband). Then, it was time to go through the egg retrieval process.

During the retrieval procedure, they put me into a twilight sleep. It turned out that the medication did its job, and the doctors were able to harvest 17 eggs. Success!

That same visit, they sent Chris to the bathroom to make his "donation," and he came back with a brown paper bag with a plastic cup inside and gave it to the lab. By this time, bodily functions were just talked about as a fact of life. Throughout the IVF process, I remember thinking that one day, I would like to have my personal privacy back.

The next step was explained to us, but we weren't prepared for the emotions that accompanied it. We were going full-speed ahead with the process of IVF, so when the sperm and eggs were put together in the petri dish in the lab, we were hoping for immediate, clear expectations such as "statistics show that 50% of eggs are fertilized." Chris asked the lab technician, "Now what?" and he said, "We wait." We took some deep breaths, waited, and prayed.

The date of conception of the embryos was February 16, 2000.

The plan was to let the embryos grow for five days, then see how many were "viable," meaning healthy and strong enough to potentially implant in my uterus. Scientists call this the "blastocyst" stage, when the embryos are dividing and creating more cells. The heaviness of waiting for five days showed us that God was in control of creating those tiny embryos…our babies. There was nothing more we could do to make anything happen. Moments like those change your perspective on the beginning of life, and nothing anyone can say will change that belief for us. We felt helpless but, with our strong faith in God, we knew that there was solid ground to stand on. During those five days, I was taking medication to prepare my uterus for implantation. The medication started building the lining of my womb up in preparation for potential pregnancy.

On day five, we found out that things had gone very well in that petri dish. We had 14 viable embryos. FOURTEEN!

Keeping in mind that I already knew we could create embryos due to the ectopic pregnancy, and I had no history of problems with my uterus, the decision was made to use two of the embryos. That meant we had a higher chance of having twins, but that was fine with us. We thought a "Buy One Get One Free" deal would be a great thing! The fertility doctors grade the embryos based on the Gardner Blastocyst Grading System, which looks at the stage of development (1-6), quality of inner mass cells(A-C), and the quality of the cells that will form the placenta(A-C). So, the doctors chose the top two "AA" embryos for implantation.

Prior to doing IVF, couples are counseled about the possibility of "extra" embryos. We did go through some counseling with Nashville Fertility Center about the possibility of producing multiple embryos and what that would be like. We knew that any additional embryos would be cryopreserved and could be used to keep expanding our family in the future. But, truthfully, that was the least of our worries at that time.

Looking back, being young and not being parents yet, it was impossible to have the long-term vision that we might need to make a decision about what to do with embryos that were not used. Couples going through fertility treatments are laser-focused on having one successful pregnancy. One baby they could call their own. One success in a sea of percentages and what-ifs.

Chris and I had discussed it at length and decided that we only wanted to go through this process once. If we were able to have twins, then we didn't want to go through the process again. I was already 33 and he was 36. If we did it again, we would be getting closer to 40.

The embryo transfer procedure happened on February 21, 2000. It was pretty quick and non-eventful, similar to visits to the gynecologist. We headed to a nearby hotel afterward, and I had to lay on my back with my legs up for several hours afterwards. I remember being afraid to move, to breathe, or go to the bathroom. After 48 hours, I was allowed to go home and resume my normal activities. My next appointment at the fertility clinic was about six weeks away. Six weeks of trying to be "normal" after two months of injections, blood draws, and lying in a prone position for various tests and procedures. I felt anything but normal.

We also found out that, of the 12 embryos that were not implanted, eight made it successfully through the cryopreservation process. The majority of them were also Grade A.

During those days, the God-given "peace that passes understanding" was with us. I just "knew that I knew that I knew" that I was pregnant. I wish that peace for anyone that goes through IVF or other infertility procedures. To know in your heart what the outcome is—positive or negative—takes away the questions and confusion. It's not just a saying that God does not give us confusion. He gives us solid answers, and no matter what that answer might be, our heart can be settled by knowing.

"For God is not a God of disorder but of peace…"(1 Corinthians 14:33)

Twins

I'm not known for being patient. I'm a Type-A, "get it done" type of person. By the time we went through IVF, I'd worked my way up to administrative positions within hospitals. So, I decided to use some leverage to find out basic information before I was scheduled to go back to the doctor in six weeks. The first indicator of pregnancy is the HCG hormone. I convinced the lab at the hospital to do an HCG test for me.

Normal pregnancy at 1-2 weeks is between 1-300. On February 28, 2000, 12 days post-conception, and seven days after implantation, my HCG count was 103. We felt confident that something good was going on in my body. We knew that at least one embryo "took." Three days later, we repeated the test, and my HCG had skyrocketed to 491.

Then, I convinced a local OB/GYN to give me an ultrasound, and we saw two sacs—twins, but still very early development. Since we had the actual conception date of the embryos, we had a day-by-day description of what was happening in the babies' growth. Between the time I had that secret ultrasound until the time for my doctor's appointment, I knew the heartbeats would start. What should I eat? Apples? Orange Juice? Chris and I had both been so involved in every tiny step of the In Vitro process, from the injections to the embryo implantation. But now that I was pregnant, we had to trust that God's plan for our babies was going to be fulfilled. I could do everything right: eat the right food, take the right vitamins, and pray the right prayers. It was daunting, and every little thing felt monumental, but God was in control.

At six weeks, just a week after the sneaky ultrasound, we had our follow-up appointment at Nashville Fertility Center. We were somewhat prepared since I had seen the two sacs already, but were still anxious about what we might find out. Sure enough: there were two heartbeats, in two separate sacs. A twin pregnancy was confirmed, and I was released from the fertility center to go back to my OB/GYN's office in Cookeville. By now, Dr. Stuber had retired, but one of Chris' high school friends, Dr. Burt Geer, was an OB/GYN in Cookeville and had twins himself. We were now considered a normal twin pregnancy.

Me? Pregnant?

Normal? We didn't have a concept of what that meant. The shock of going through complicated fertility tests, surgery, treatments and then IVF was not considered normal. I had not thought much about morning sickness, maternity clothes, or even learning to change a diaper.

Being pregnant was a concept I didn't think was possible. *I'm not supposed to be pregnant...I can't get pregnant.* I had coped with my situation by believing for many years that I was unable to bear my own children and that we would probably end up adopting at least one child.

That had been the conversation for many years, with well-meaning friends saying, "just quit trying and it will just happen," not realizing that I had no fallopian tubes and that it wasn't going to "just happen." Eventually, I'd respond with a smile and a nod. It was just too complicated and exhausting to explain.

Even while pregnant, I still related to women with fertility issues. Even today, I still feel a deep connection with women who struggle with infertility. My heart aches for those who feel like science experiments and are poked, prodded, and stuck with needles in order to achieve what others can do multiple times before they reach the age of thirty. I did feel blessed that we had a path to fertility shown to us since I had the ectopic pregnancy. But I always have carried "survival guilt" that I was able to achieve pregnancy when others have not.

Another big moment was finding out the gender of the babies. Since we were having two babies, and I'm a planner, I didn't want any surprises. When the babies were big enough to tell gender, it was VERY obvious on the ultrasound…two "turtle heads" made it very clear I was carrying two boys. We went from the doctor's office to the drug store, bought two blue bows and stuck them on my tummy, then went to my mom's house to tell her the news. Not much of a gender reveal, but we had enough surprises, so it was fun to start planning with lots of blue.

Deciding names for Baby A and Baby B was pretty easy. Chris's full name is Christopher Matthew Martin. So, Baby A was named Christopher, and Baby B was named Matthew. We decided that their middle names needed to have some historical significance. My father's name is Robert, and I thought it flowed well with Matthew, so Baby B's full name became Matthew Robert Martin. Before Chris was born, his mom lost a baby at only a few months from suspected crib death. That baby was Scotty, and after Scotty died his parents decided to have one more baby, who was Chris. So, we decided to name Baby A Christopher Scott Martin.

During the IVF process and the pregnancy, our church family was praying and supporting us. I have memories of going to the altar at church and thanking God for all He had done for me and our marriage in such a short time. Jason Yarbrough's wife, Susan, told me once that she felt gratitude radiating from me. I was reminded how I told God I wanted "proof" in Him and in the story of Jesus. The proof was all around me, in my heart, and with those two baby boys kicking inside my womb.

A twin pregnancy is not usually routine, but other than a couple of minor trips to the doctor and two overnight stays in the hospital to monitor Braxton-Hicks contractions, my pregnancy was very uneventful. I was very sick for the first two-three months, and then I was VERY large. My mother said when I was pregnant and walked into a room, I filled the entire space and turned lots of heads. We took a trip to San Diego, California when I was about five months along, and I craved the hottest habanero salsa all day—from my scrambled eggs in the morning to the fajitas at dinner. I had many people ask, "When are you due?" and when I responded, "Not for four months," the shock on their faces was apparent. I looked nine months pregnant when I was around five months with the twins.

We also had to make several life changes during those days so that I could even function. I'd been driving a cute little red Eagle Talon, and by seven months, I simply could not fit in it. Chris had also just bought a beautiful cream-colored Ford F150 King Cab truck that he loved. But we traded in that truck for a minivan, and Chris drove the Talon.

We had been married 12 years at that point, and we had always slept on a waterbed. Originally, we used the one that Chris had—the relic 1980s waterbed that could catapult someone off one side if the other person sat down hard enough on the opposite side. Over the years, we had invested in a more modern waterbed that had fibers which provided more support than the original one. But now, getting in and out of that bed required a two-person assist. So, the waterbed had to go, and a regular bed with a box spring and mattress was the replacement.

I had a beautiful baby shower that my mother orchestrated for friends and family, and another one that the church gave me. We chose a Noah's Ark theme for the nursery and the showers. A woman from our church made an incredible Noah's Ark cake that matched the baby quilts we had chosen for the nursery. It was such a joyous time, with so much support from friends and family. And the amount of baby toys, clothes, accessories, and equipment was incredible. Two of nearly everything! My artist mother spent hours painting a mural of Noah's Ark on the nursery wall that also matched the nursery theme. Chris was tasked with putting together 2 cribs and finding room in the nursery and in our house for all of the gifts. There were so many items that were recommended to make raising twin babies easier, and one of those was a double stroller. We received the double stroller we requested at one of the baby showers, and we used it for years, learning to transfer the two baby carriers from the stroller to the minivan and then using it for the boys to sit in when they grew into toddlers.

I kept working until I was 32 weeks pregnant; then I became too big to be productive. I gained a total of 80 pounds and also craved Sonic Peanut Butter sundaes. At 34 weeks, Dr. Geer said the boys were both developed enough to be safely born. The Braxton Hicks contractions had stopped, but I thought I would go into labor by 35 weeks. There was no mention of inducing labor since many twin pregnancies don't go over 35-37 weeks. But my boys were stubborn.

On Sunday, October 15, 2000, we went to church then decided to go to Waffle House, which was the extent of what I could manage with my reduced energy level at that time. We walked into the restaurant and went to a booth, soon to realize that I couldn't fit in it. We had to find a random chair to pull up to the side of the booth so I could eat with my husband. I was so ready to have the babies.

At 37 weeks, on October 17, (two days after the Waffle House incident), the water in Christopher's sac broke in the middle of the night, and we were off to Cookeville General Hospital, about a 30-minute drive from our house. I had everything already packed and ready to go, but we had heard so many stories about labor happening fast and babies born in the car on the way to the hospital. So, we hurried and sped in the dark in the minivan in those early hours to get there. However, my body didn't go into labor easily, so after 12 hours of waiting, I was given Pitocin, which was not a good experience. My body was under such duress that I would fall asleep between contractions, then wake up and focus on my friend Eileen, who had agreed to be there with me during the labor process. She had given birth to three boys of her own, was an amazing Christian woman, and had such a calming presence. Chris was there holding my hand and reminding me to breathe and focus.

The plan all along was to go ahead and give me an epidural because more than likely I was going to have a C-section. Dr. Geer was returning from a family vacation that day, and his estimated time of arrival was sometime in the evening of the 17th. However, the anesthesiologist who was on call that day had apparently done some recent research that convinced him he needed to wait until I was at least five centimeters dilated to give me that epidural. Throughout the next few hours, my husband had heated discussions with the anesthesiologist because I was experiencing painful contractions in waves and was having trouble dilating to five cm. By the time Dr. Geer arrived on the scene around 8PM, he could see that I was in distress and literally looked at me, peeked underneath the sheet and declared "she's five cm—give her the epidural!"

Once the epidural was given, my body relaxed and within 5 hours I was able to attempt a natural delivery. Repeat, ATTEMPT a natural delivery, because after pushing for two hours I saw the nurses' eyes peeking out from above their surgical masks with looks of concern. The boys were stuck with Christopher head down and Matthew spread-eagle across the top, filling my ribcage. Chris says that he could see Christopher's head trying to come out, but then it would go back in. After a short discussion during which I made it very clear that I was ready to move to the next option, I was prepped for a C-section.

Christopher Scott Martin and Matthew Robert Martin were born three minutes apart, the morning of October 18, 2000. Christopher weighed 5 lb, 8 oz and Matthew weighed 7 lb 0 oz. Yep, almost 13 pounds of baby! I barely remember the event. I was exhausted and woozy. No neonatal intensive care, no issues—two healthy baby boys.

But I do remember Chris trying to make a joke, saying "Matthew is perfect other than he has six toes." Yes, he said that, and I was not amused.

Immediately after their birth, I discovered the maternal connection that everyone talks about. The boys were born around 4 AM on Wednesday, so I needed time to recover. Sleep was precious. It would be years before I would get a solid night's sleep again, and it all started in the hospital. Every time I woke up and called the nursery to check on the "twinkies," as they were nicknamed by the nurses, the response was ALWAYS: "Actually, Christopher just woke up!" There was something sweet and magical about that, until it became annoying. My sweet little Christopher, who I adore to this day, did not let me sleep a single night for at least two years.

Five days later they sent us home. We were terrified. Don't some people leave their babies in the care of the nurses for a few more days? We needed just a couple of days to sleep! We remember even struggling to make sure that both of the carriers were "clicked" into the car base correctly. We were both exhausted. But the heartburn I had for the past three months was finally gone, so on the way home we went to the Burger King drive thru and I got a double cheeseburger.

We brought the babies in the two carriers in the house, sat them down in the foyer, and said, *"Now what do we do"*?

That's a reality check that many couples face when going through infertility treatments then bringing home a baby. So much energy, emotion, and focus goes into bringing those babies healthy into the world. The day-to-day work of two babies didn't work its way into my mindset until late in my pregnancy.

It was a shock.

No sleep and an embryo decision

The next year was more hectic than I could have ever imagined. There were two sets of EVERYTHING—diapers, bottles, formula, pacifiers. The sleep deprivation was overwhelming, and I became obsessed trying to create order out of chaos. Getting the twins on the same schedule of eating, playing and sleeping was challenging but was my way of survival. I was unable to get the hang of nursing the boys simultaneously, so I devised a method of feeding them at the same time. I would sit on the floor with my back to a chair or couch, have one baby nursing and holding him with one arm, then the other in a bouncy chair on the floor. The baby in the bouncy would take a bottle, then the next time they would switch places.

The worst part about this arrangement was that my body was only producing enough milk for one baby. So, between feeding them every two to three hours, I would also pump to provide enough milk. This schedule was round the clock. It exhausted me, and I became so insensitive to the process that I would just lift my shirt and hook up the pump, no matter who was visiting.

I remember being motivated by a friend of mine named Tammy. She had gone through IVF, and the doctors implanted two embryos, then one split and she had triplets—two identical boys and a girl. She was also an RN and lactation consultant, and she nursed those babies for over a year. I could not even imagine having triplets!

Chris took a few weeks off work and had to get up early to be at Pizza Hut at 7AM, so he handled the early morning feeding to let me sleep. He did everything from changing diapers, cleaning bottles, and telling me "it will all be OK."

My mother loved the twins and wanted to be a typical grandma; she wanted to rock and hold them. But I needed someone to do the heavy work. Taking care of twins was more work than I ever thought I could handle, and it was definitely more than my mother could handle on her own. The boys were a month old when the Christmas season started, and my mother wanted to put up a Christmas tree. I honestly didn't care if we had a Christmas tree or any decorations. I needed sleep and clean laundry.

In the middle of this phase of no sleep, 10-12 diapers a day, kitchen sinks full of bottles, and pumping every three hours, the Nashville Fertility Center checked in with us to see if we wanted to keep the embryos frozen, or use them, or consider other options.

My first thought was: *Are you serious?*

Christopher was colicky, and Matthew wanted to sleep all the time. I couldn't even imagine having more babies. Matthew had trouble with formula and projectile vomited when he was burped. We had a dog named Bart—a dachshund who had his world rocked when we brought home two babies. Now, when I was burping Matthew and my other hand was full with Christopher, Bart would wait for the projectile milk to hit the carpet and then lick it up. My life was incredibly different, and they wanted me to decide if I wanted more babies?

It was February, 2001, almost a year since conception. Cryopreservation is paid by the year, so when the boys were only a few months old, we revisited our decision to only go through IVF one time and be happy with what God decided to give us. Plus, I didn't want eight more babies, or to have twins again—or even triplets.

The options were to:

1) keep the embryos frozen indefinitely,
2) use the embryos,
3) donate them to science,
4) let them thaw out, or
5) give them a chance by donating them back to the fertility clinic for other couples to potentially adopt.

The choice was clear from the moment we looked at the options. I knew that the kind of person who would use someone else's embryos to get pregnant, bear the children, and raise them as their own had to have a special heart. She would probably not be able to get pregnant on her own and would want to have that experience so badly that she would be willing to go through a similar process that I went through to have an embryo implanted. Then, she would have to know that the baby was biologically not hers but still allow her blood to run through the umbilical cord to bond with that baby. Then she would love that baby as her own, knowing in her heart that one day they might know their biological history.

That mother would have to be a very caring, loving, accepting person.

Honestly, I'm not sure I am the kind of woman who could have done that. My need as a woman was not necessarily to be pregnant, and I would have been OK if we had to adopt a baby.

On March 26, 2001, we officially donated our eight precious embryos to the Nashville Fertility Center. Once we donated the embryos, we understood that there would be no connection to them, and we would give up any ability to ever find out what happened to them. It was considered a donation of property. Legally, they weren't considered babies, but we knew they were.

We filled out the forms about our education, lifestyle, belief systems, health background and other family history, and it was done.

Over the years, I always wondered—prayed—I even bargained with God wondering what I could do to prove myself strong enough to know what happened to those babies. But faith in God has a way of settling even the most anxious momma's heart, just like He did for Mary when she seemed to know that there was something special about her son.

"And Mary kept all these things, pondering them in her heart." Luke 2:19

"And his (Jesus') mother treasured up all these things in her heart." Luke 2:51

God had those babies in the palm of his hand, and I knew that I would probably never know what happened to them. I had to learn to be OK with that. I had learned that "faith is the evidence of things unseen." I knew faith had to be my strength.

There was one time that I remember wondering if I should have gone back and used more of the embryos—gone through IVF one more time. Maybe I had made a mistake? The boys were under two years old, and I actually contacted the clinic about it. They said I would have to go through counseling again, and it was a complicated process. Our deciding factor on not going through IVF again was two-fold. If I "un-donated," I would know if any of them had been used. I realized that if I found out, I couldn't un-learn that information. I would have to live with it, and I wasn't ready for that information. The other factor was that even if I used two or three of the embryos, there would STILL be more frozen, and I would STILL wonder what happened to them. So, we decided to look to the future, continue to trust God with the fate of the embryos, and raise our little family.

Being a stay-at-home mom

The first two years of the boys' lives were in Sparta, Tennessee. Although I had a corporate job that I loved, I was overcome with a sudden, strong God-given craving to be home with my babies. We tried several different daycare situations—even Chris' niece for a short time. I was a stickler for keeping a schedule. One daycare I used decided to ignore my instructions to wake up sleepy-head Matthew when Christopher woke up so they could eat at the same time. This created a chaotic popcorn schedule for my evenings and nights, each waking up separately, sometimes within 30 mins to an hour of each other. It was truly one of the most trying times in my life, and I experienced some post-partum depression. I was surviving day-to-day, and I was too tired to envision that life wouldn't always be that way. One of my husband's favorite sayings during those first months was "the sun will always come up tomorrow." There were days that saying truly kept me going.

 I was trying to work my corporate job but living on very little sleep, which was affecting my performance. I was also driving a 45-minute commute over Bonair Mountain from Sparta to Crossville every day. There were times that I cried all the way to work. I missed my babies, and juggling my work and home schedules was taking a toll on me both mentally and physically.

 Before becoming pregnant, I was a pretty fit person. I like to work out and eat healthy—no carbs and very little caffeine. But now, I needed caffeine to function and ate junk food in my car. No one told me life would change SO MUCH after having twins.

 I decided that being a stay-at-home mom was the only way that my heart, spirit and body was going to be able to survive. Let me reword that: God decided. I was miserable without my babies! But we always had lived off two incomes and truly didn't know how we would be able to survive financially if I didn't work. We had a fairly new home along with a mortgage, plus the cost of diapers, food and supplies for two babies. I sat down and had a heart-to-heart with my boss. The company had seen me through the changes over the past few years, including the IVF process, so I was sad to leave. But he was very understanding and also agreed that the quality of my work was suffering. The company let me draw unemployment for a while, which helped cover the bills.

 And once again, God provided. He loves His children and

makes things happen that we cannot fathom. That pivot was February 2001, and the boys were four months old.

A month after I decided to be a stay-at-home mom, Chris called from work saying he had hurt his neck cleaning a pizza oven. He went to the orthopedic doctor who ordered him to stay home, not lift anything, and draw worker's compensation. So, there we were... me on unemployment and Chris drawing worker's compensation. Two healthy incomes to zero in a matter of a month, and Chris couldn't lift our two babies who were still immobile and in carriers.

"*Ok God...is THIS what it's going to be?*" I asked. We were still flying high on our newfound faith and all that God had done for us, and we found support and comfort from our church family. But there was no hiding the fact that it was HARD.

In fact, we thought it would be impossible.

Even though we had been through miracles over the past two years, there we were being our stubborn selves and thinking that things couldn't possibly work. The bills had to be paid, and my meticulous Excel spreadsheet told me that we would be in the red very quickly.

Within a few weeks of Chris' neck injury, it was apparent that he needed surgery to clean out some vertebrae in his upper neck that had been damaged while he was reaching into the large pizza ovens and lifting heavy pans and racks. The surgery was very invasive, and he required pain medicine on a regular schedule, including Oxycodone. This was 2001, before there was widespread knowledge on the addictive powers of opioids. So, just as the doctor ordered, I made sure that Chris had his pain under control every four-six hours. A few weeks later, he decided to switch to Tylenol because the healing was going well. Within 12 hours, he felt like he was getting the flu. Nausea, sweating, and shaking badly. We called the doctor who informed us that the Oxycodone was very addictive, and he should not stop taking it cold turkey. No one had told us that when the drug was prescribed. So, he started tapering off the Oxycodone with the reminder to NEVER use that again if at all possible.

Just a month later, in May 2001, I celebrated my first Mother's

Day as a mom. My amazing church family gave me the chance to tell my story of redemption and motherhood in the pulpit that Sunday. I was so excited and nervous; so many of these people had seen Chris and I get saved, become an active member of the church, pray through the In Vitro process, and now were helping raise our family. I shared our story along with pictures of Christopher and Matthew as five day old embryos—then as newborn babies! I also included our decision about embryo donation, letting them know that God had made it clear that those embryos were our babies and that I trusted Him to take care of them, although I would never know the outcome.

But our concerns at that point were focused on Chris's recuperation and figuring out how to pay the bills. I was still at home caring for the boys and had help from friends and family. Each month that passed I would declare, "Next month I'm going to have to go back to work," because the numbers on our budget did not match up due to our suddenly-dropped income. But each month came and somehow we paid our bills, bought diapers, and baby food. Each month the reliance on our faith was tested and proved. In addition to receiving anonymous monetary gifts, I utilized the WIC (Women, Infants and Children) program and learned to make money stretch.

When Moses led the captives to freedom across the Red Sea, God told them to build a monument out of 12 stones so they could come back and be reminded of what God had done. He had done the impossible…changed Pharoah's heart AND parted the sea! What did they do? In just a short period of time... THEY FORGOT! Their forgetfulness and lack of faith left them wandering in the desert for 40 years before reaching their promised land. And here we were with two miracle babies—thinking that God was out of the miracle business. We were, and still are, so human, and we are so in need of God's mercy and grace. We didn't know that He was going to remind us again in a big way how reliable He is.

By July of 2001, Chris was still recuperating and was not back at work yet. His doctors encouraged him to consider another job that wouldn't have him doing as much manual labor. But we were in a small town, with family around, and Chris couldn't imagine how he could find another line of work.

While waiting to be medically released, my friend Cheri asked, "Doesn't Chris get a remuneration for his worker's comp injury?" Honestly, we hadn't thought about it. We checked with a worker's comp attorney and sure enough there was a process that figured out a monetary settlement for worker's compensation injuries. We were limping financially, and every month I repeated the belief that I would need to find employment again soon, even if Chris went back to work.

After waiting several months to find out the financial settlement, we received a worker's compensation check on December 31, 2001. We were able to pay off everything except our mortgage, and we ceremoniously burned all of our bills in our fireplace. We consider this one of the times we built a monument to remember what God did for us. This method of being out of debt is NOT recommended. Chris suffered so much and it was a very hard time for us. But God chose this path, we believe, to build our faith. From then on, and for six years, I was a stay-at-home mom with my two rambunctious, busy, hysterical and adorable twin boys. But the last of Chris' injuries was still ahead of us.

Not again!

During my time staying home in Sparta, we went to Nashville several times to see my childhood friend Joanna. We'd been inseparable since 1st grade, so it was very special being able to visit "Aunt Joanna." We would take the babies to malls in the double stroller, and I always loved stopping to encourage other twin moms and ask about their journey. If I ever saw someone with triplets, I would stop and praise them for the incredible job they are doing in just surviving. I never considered the fact that one of those twin or triplet moms could have my biological children in their stroller. Honestly, the reality that someone else could be pregnant with or giving birth to our biological children so soon after our boys were born didn't occur to me. Maybe I thought that God would wait awhile to let things settle. Maybe I thought he had done enough miracles that he was taking a break. I was so incredibly clueless and lost in my haze of raising my sons.

In the fall of 2002, it happened again. Chris was doing some heavy lifting at work, and his vertebrae gave out. It was the same one that caused the trouble the last time, but now it was worse. The vertebrae had slipped out of place and it needed to be fused.

Again God? Really?

The boys were two years old and very busy toddlers. But by this time, our faith had been strengthened, fortified by trials we had gone through those first years. The surgery went well, and Chris declared that he would not get addicted to Oxycodone, although he might need it for a short time.

I have to admit, I was scared. This was a much more invasive surgery, which included removal of bone. I imagined the pain must be intense, and I didn't want Chris to suffer. Eight days after surgery, with daily use of Oxycodone, as we were on our way to church, I reminded him that it was time to take his pain meds. Chris said, "I'm not taking them today." I was very worried that we would get to church and the sweats and shaking would start. I watched him carefully all during the service, and by noon I realized he wasn't having symptoms. We went out to lunch and came home—and still no sweating, no nausea, and no shaking.

I said to him, "Chris… you have been healed of that addiction!"

We both praised God for that.

However, the problem of his job became more prevalent. Our friend Ron was a family practice doctor, and he spoke very sternly to Chris that he really needed to find a different line of work, because this type of injury would very likely keep happening if he kept doing heavy labor. In addition, this was the second worker's compensation injury at his job as a Pizza Hut Manager. The fear of losing his job crossed his mind many times, and he still hadn't been given the clearance to go back to work by March 2003.

At the beginning of April 2003, Chris got a message that his regional director wanted to talk to him. We were fully prepared that he might be fired from his job. How many companies would keep an employee who kept getting injured?

We had taken our eye off that monument we had built to remind us of God's miraculous power. But God didn't forget. He was still working on His plan.

Chris' regional director told him that there was a position open for a district manager. No lifting or heavy labor, just using his management skills to oversee operations of several Pizza Huts. They would even pay our mortgage until our house was sold. The location was Colorado Springs, Colorado.

"They are giving you a promotion?" I exclaimed. "Looks like we are moving to Colorado!"

As a young couple rebuilding our lives as new Christians with two babies, we were actually excited about the move and decided it would be an adventure. Our families were not quite as thrilled, but they also saw the miracles that were unfolding for us, and they supported us in our decision. My mother declared that she would visit regularly. Chris' mother had passed away the year before, and his father had moved to Florida. So, the timing of the move seemed to work.

We made the move to the mountains of Colorado in June 2003.

Busy days in Colorado

Colorado Springs was a great place to raise a family. It was a conservative town with lots of good churches, two military bases—Fort Carson Army Base and Peterson Air Force Base—and the Air Force Academy. Chris' job as a district manager for Pizza Hut meant he had to travel overnight quite a bit. He traveled between Limon, Colorado, in the far east part of the state, all the way to Grand Junction in the west part. Sometimes snow storms would hit in the high country, and he would get stuck in Breckenridge on the west side of the Eisenhower Tunnel and be unable to drive home. Being at home with the boys was fun but truly exhausting. To keep my brain functioning and doing something creative, I started scrapbooking. I would stay up until midnight putting together pages of photos, and I would handwrite fonts that would fit the mood of the pages.

There were several times Chris and I loaded up the boys and joined in Chris' trips to the high country of Colorado. We have many memories of snowmobiling, exploring cowboy towns, and seeing the tourist sites.

We also found a church home—Friendship Assembly of God—and became very involved. The church was an Assembly of God church with solid conservative values—similar to Trinity Assembly but much smaller. The days we spent learning the basics of the Christian faith at Trinity Assembly proved essential in finding a church that had the same values. Christopher and Matthew were well loved by the congregation, the children's pastor and Sunday school teachers. One teacher in particular was a woman who must have been in her 70's. We could tell she had the ability to discipline and call out disruptive behavior, and in one instance she pulled us aside and told us that Christopher was "throwing his colors" in Sunday school and that she had put him in a corner in time out. She was a hoot. Thank God for our church families over the years!

Several times during those years in Colorado, we would come back to Tennessee to visit family. Chris' company even had a big event at the Opryland Hotel in 2004. We brought the boys, and they stayed with family for part of the time, and we also spent some time in Nashville showing our then 4-year-olds some sites in Nashville.

During those years in Colorado, we also met some amazing friends. Missy and Mike Mire lived around the corner from us and were from Louisiana. Mike was in the Air Force and was a bigger-than-life Loo-siana personality, and Missy cooked the best Cajun food I have ever eaten. They were also an incredible Christian couple that helped support us when the boys were at their most rambunctious. We spent many Sunday afternoons in their LSU-purple painted basement watching football, praying together for our families, and leaning on each other when her kids were teenagers and mine were toddlers. When the call came that they were being relocated to Wichita Falls, Texas, I was incredibly sad. The boys would soon be starting kindergarten, and I was coming out of my five-year fog of having twins.

There was a new charter school opening close to where we

lived in southeast Colorado Springs, and we were lucky enough to have the boys selected from a lottery to attend. The first day of kindergarten, I took the boys to their classroom and looked around at all of the other moms who were generally five to ten years younger than me. Many were going to work out, meeting friends or doing active things while their kids were in kindergarten. I just wanted to take a nap. While standing in line to meet the teacher, I started talking to another woman who looked to be about my age. She had two beautiful little girls with her—a blonde ray of sunshine named Alissa, who was in the same class as Christopher and Matthew, and a tiny brunette fireball named Jenna, who was only about a year younger than her big sister. From that moment on, De and I became best friends. When I found out that her girls were both adopted, I appreciated her even more.

The big test was having our husbands meet, so we set up a dinner double date. De's husband, Jeff, was so happy to be around other boys, and I was so happy to be around other girls! We believe our friendship was set up by God, and we are best friends to this day. They were originally from San Antonio and continually talked about how great Texas is.

We lived in Colorado for six-and-a-half years, spending many evenings and weekends with the Marshalls and letting the kids run rampant. I took a job at the corporate office of Community Bible Study as the National Training Coordinator, and De was a real estate agent. Many times we would pick up each other's kids from school and meet at one of our houses, then hang out for dinner. Our husbands had to ask which house we landed at so they knew where to show up.

After a few years, Chris got tired of traveling and found another job that would allow him to be home more. But in 2007, when the boys were in 2nd grade, Chris suddenly lost his job. There were not many jobs available in Colorado Springs, but I believed we were supposed to stay there.

After two months of job hunting, one of Chris' old bosses contacted him about a job opening in Tucson, Arizona. I rolled my eyes and said "YOU go to Tucson. I'm staying here." After all, we had Jeff and De, and we were supposed to raise our kids together. My job was at a Christian organization. Life was good, and apparently God didn't get the memo that I had planned out my entire life.

Through anger and tears, I called our pastor's wife and told her about our situation. I was praying for doors to open for a job in Colorado, and it seemed like it wasn't happening and was causing strife between me and Chris. She gave me some of the most profound advice I have ever had in my life. She said that instead of praying for doors to open, I should pray for doors to close. So, I did.

Within days, every local job that Chris applied for turned him down. The job in Tucson was the only option. God spoke to me in my heart, telling me that I needed to be a grown-up and "put on my big girl pants," for lack of a better description. As a mother and wife, it was my job to set the mood for my family. If I was miserable, my family would be miserable.

Pivot!

I decided to attack our move as an adventure. It was a hard move for everyone since the boys were going into 2nd grade. But we leaned on our faith, believing that God had already gone before us and had planned our future. We spent three years in Arizona and had several fun vacations in Rocky Point, Mexico, which is the "local's" beach in Puerto Penasco, only four hours from our home in Tucson. We bought a 29-foot travel trailer (because I'm not a camping-in-a-tent person), and we even went to The Grand Canyon. Jeff and De and the girls visited us several times in Arizona, and we also drove back to Colorado to visit the mountains.

Being a "boy mom" was in full swing when we lived in Colorado and Arizona. I had friends with little girls, and I realized while spending time with them that it is SO DIFFERENT than raising boys. Christopher and Matthew were always on the move and loved doing anything involving speed, guns (even pretend ones), and dirt. I can't imagine having a girl to raise, and I knew that God meant this life for me.

But within three years, my longing to live back in the south took over. I missed the grass, trees, lakes, southern food, and southern hospitality. The boys were soon starting middle school (6th grade), so Chris and I started applying for jobs in the southern United States: Tennessee, Mississippi, Alabama, Texas. We decided that the first one who got the best job in the South would be the winner.

Fairly soon, I landed a job in Kingwood, Texas, on the northeast side of Houston. I was so excited. Texas had lakes and even a beach in Galveston where we could take the boys, and the food choices were phenomenal! With two growing boys, food was pretty important to us. And of course, Jeff and De always raved about how amazing Texas was.

In June of 2012 we made the trip with the two kids and our dachshund in a Ford F-150, pulling the 29-foot camping trailer from Tucson to Kingwood. We stopped in Kerrville and went fishing and had Texas BBQ. We immediately loved the state.

Within a few weeks, the boys also settled into Texas and started making friends. I knew this is where we would stay.

Twin talents and hobbies

Our boys developed different talents and hobbies over the years. Both played T-ball, football, and band in Elementary and Junior High.

Christopher was a little more on the high-strung side like me; we noticed early that he was in tune with rhythm and loved music. He would use anything he could to create noise. When he was five years old in Colorado Springs, a neighbor was selling a kid's drum set—a nice one made of metal, not plastic, so he couldn't damage it. Christopher took to the drums instantly and had all four limbs going at once! It was his outlet. While in Colorado, he played drums at school talent shows and at church. In Arizona, the boys started a band with some friends, with Christopher on drums and Matthew playing bass.

In Texas, Christopher joined the choir in sixth grade. We went to his first performance where he had a surprise solo and belted out "Chim Chimmeny" from Mary Poppins, with a voice we had never heard before. He still continued to play drums, but from then on, his vocal talent grew.

Matthew took to hands-on things like projects, yard work, and sports. He was a hard worker and got satisfaction from getting his hands dirty. From an early age he also had a very caring heart and became the "dad" of any friend group, with many girls talking to him on the phone about their problems until late into the night.

In ninth grade, the boys both went on mission trips with our church. Matthew went to Africa, and we have pictures of him playing with adorable little kids there. He always attracted children and loved them, too. Christopher went to Seattle, Washington, on his mission trip and came back with lots of lifelong memories.

Along the way, Christopher and Matthew had grown into themselves. We always told them that, although they are twins, God made them each unique, and they are not expected to have the same interests or talents.

In high school, Christopher's music talent had blossomed into many performances utilizing his unique rustic, tenor voice, his talent for drums, and now his self-taught guitar skills. He landed gigs playing at local restaurants around Houston, where he honed his skills as an amazing musician. He was known as our choir kid, excelling at state competitions in vocals as a tenor. His biggest joy, though, was leading worship at church. He truly had a talent that I described as "seeing music in 3D."

Matthew excelled in football and in the high school's Marine Junior ROTC. In high school, he had to choose between the two, and football won out. The team from his 6A Texas High School had produced several college and NFL players, and since we were in Texas, where football is king, our weekends turned into a juggle of football and choir.

My husband became well-known for his cooking, so during home game weekends we would have the offensive line from the football team over for barbecue. At the same time, several choir kids would be at our house hanging out.

Combining worlds—the yin and yang of high school—it was a fun time!

From the time the boys were in elementary school we told them that "God chose them specially to be brothers and twins." When they were old enough to know the birds and the bees, we told them the story of their conception and that there might be other siblings. I continued to give some presentations at women's and church groups about our story, showing pictures of my twins as five-day-old embryos, then as newborn babies. I would also talk about the remaining frozen embryos and how we hoped they were OK, and that we trusted that God was taking care of their precious lives.

For all those years, we repeatedly said that all we hoped for was to know that at least some of them had survived, and if any of them ever knocked on our door, we would say, "We are so glad you're alive!" We would never expect a relationship, because I wanted to respect the parents and never interfere.

But God's sovereignty would once again be shown.

Brooke Martin

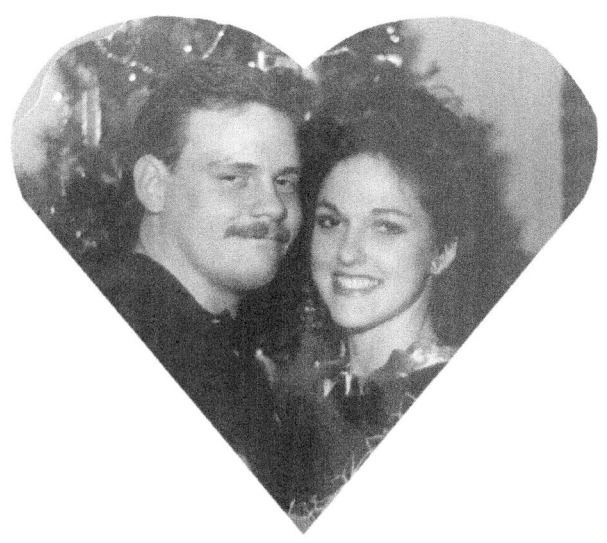

Engaged, December 1986.

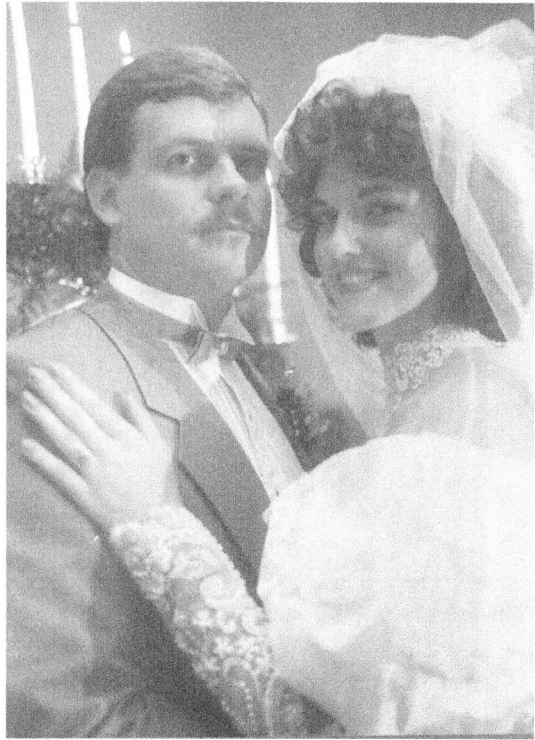

The Big Wedding, July 25, 1987.

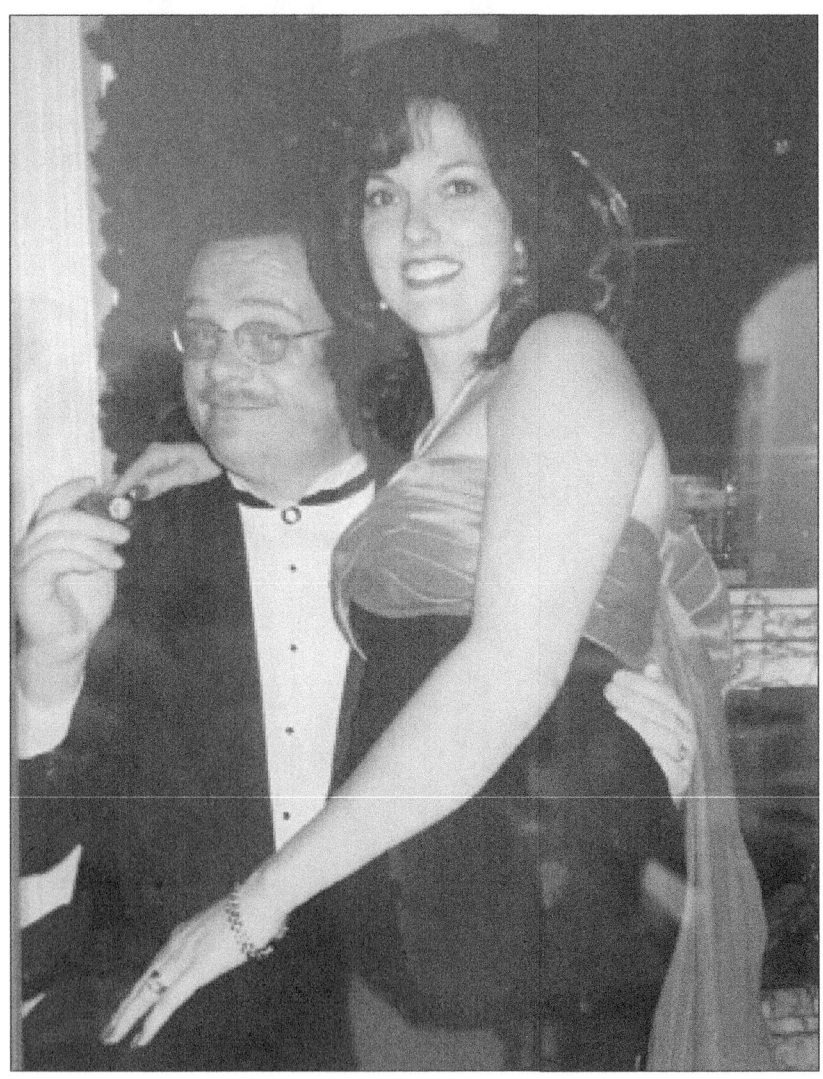

New Year in New Orleans, Mid 1990s.

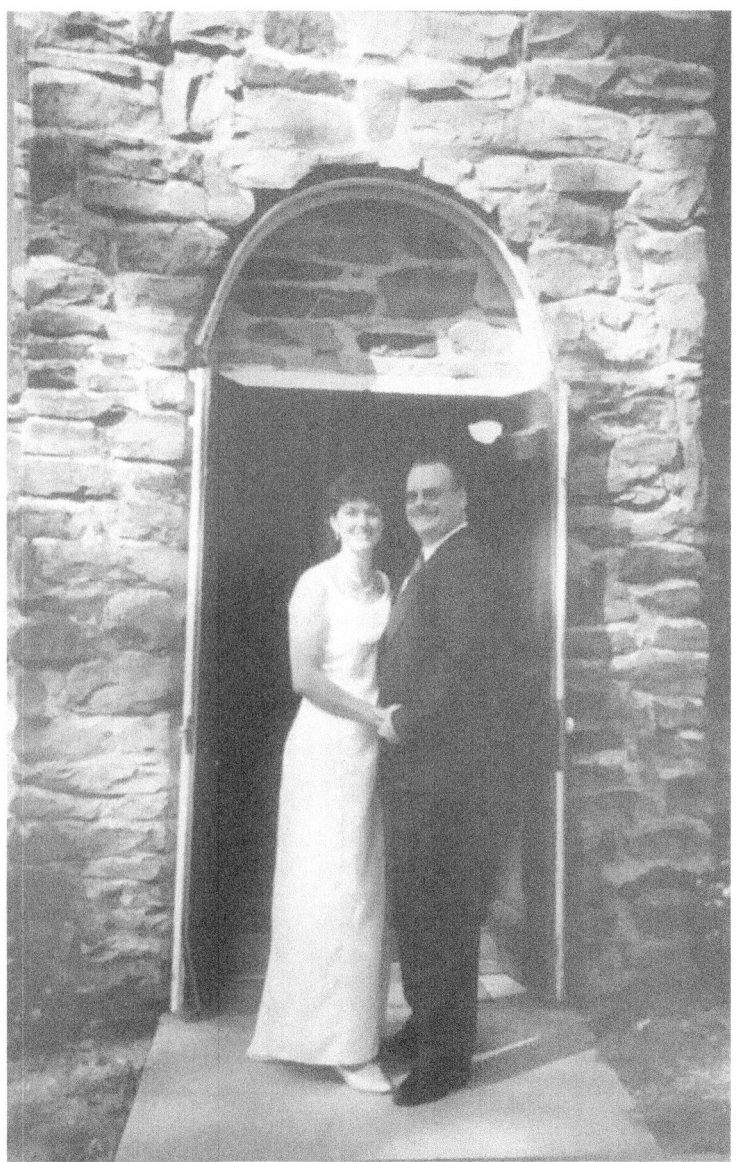

Renewing our vows, September 25, 1999.

Our Love Multiplied

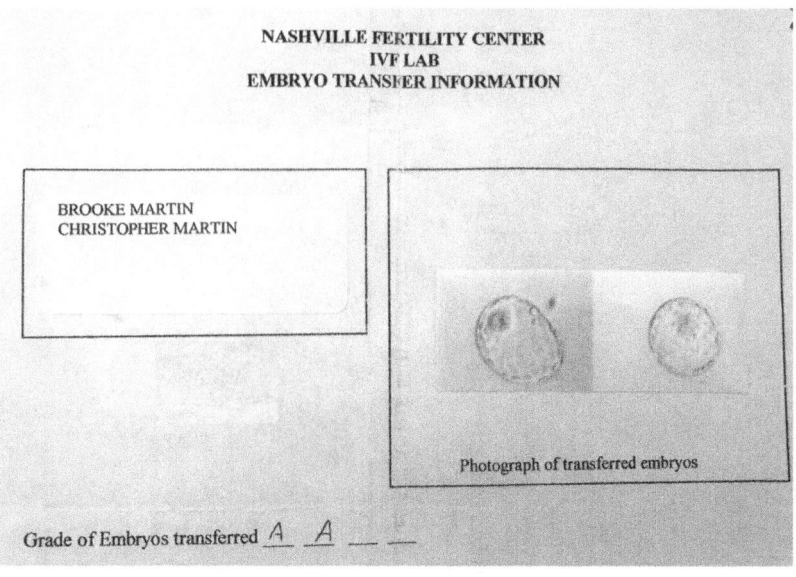

The two, 5-day-old embryos that were transferred (Christopher and Matthew Martin).

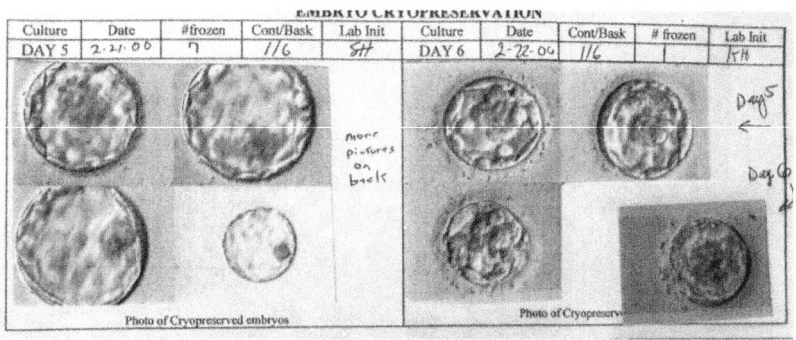

The eight embryos that were cryopreserved.

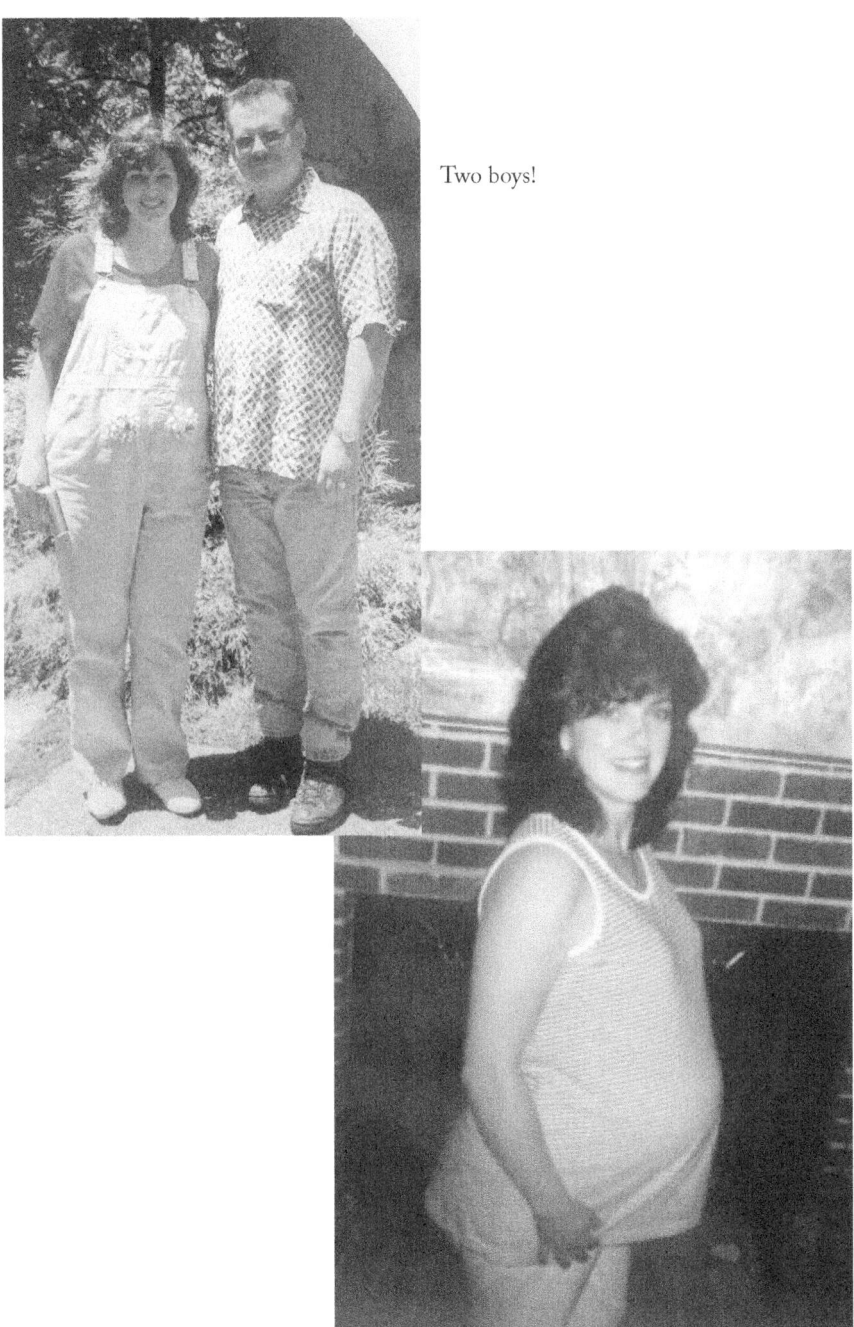

Two boys!

Six months pregnant with twins.

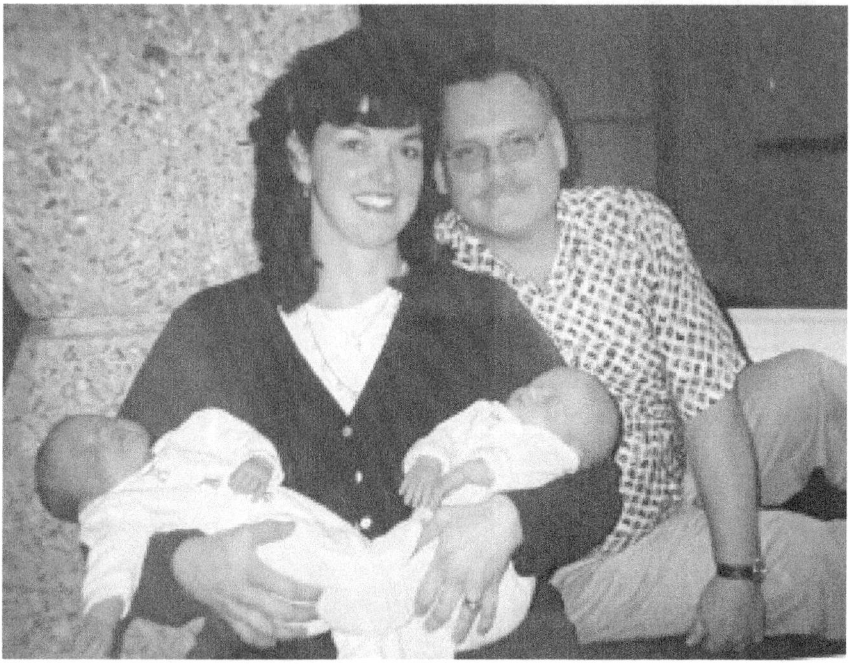

Our Love Multiplied

Chris and Brooke with newborns Matthew (L) and Christopher (R).

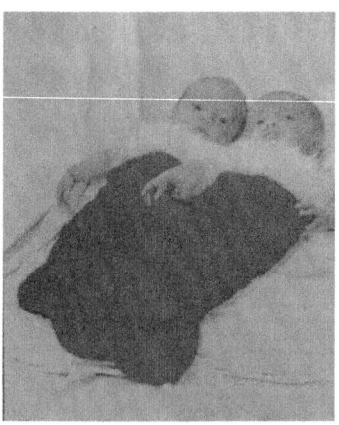

Our Christmas Stockings, Dec. 2000.

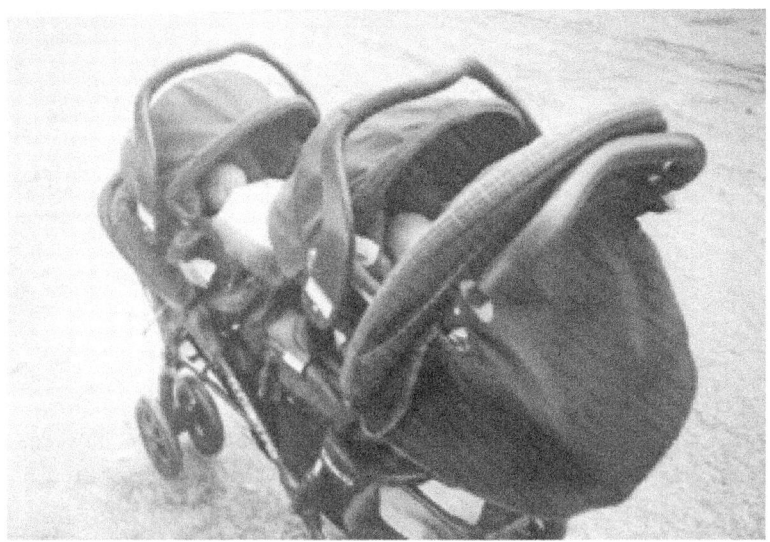

The double stroller.

Christopher riding on Matthew's back, age 2.

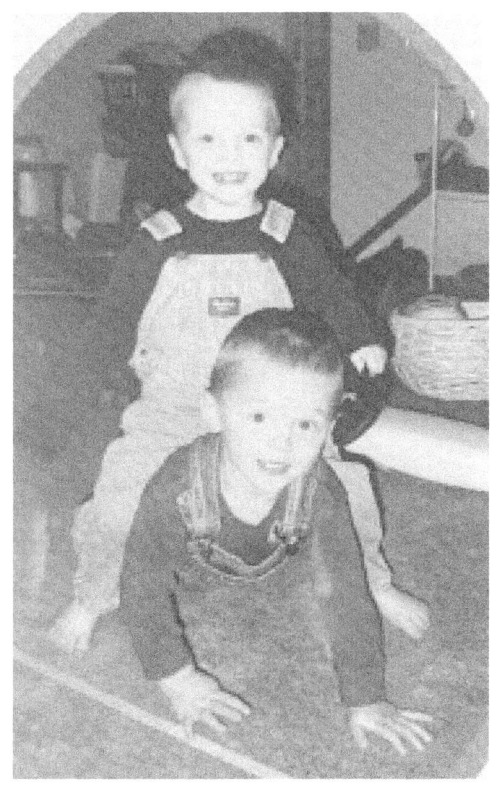

Our Love Multiplied

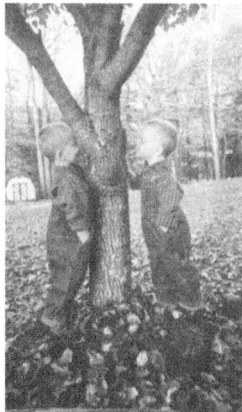

Peek-a-boo boys, age 2.

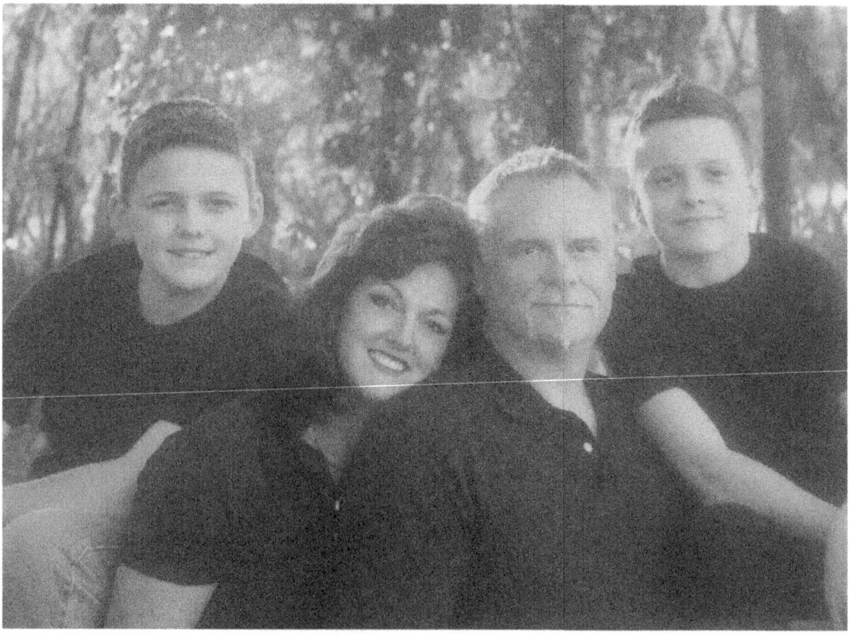

(L-R) Matthew, Brooke, Chris, and Christopher after our move to Texas in 2013.

Part 2—The Connection

The call

In 2021, I had the biggest pivot of my life. It was the call that my husband and I thought we might get someday, but we still weren't prepared.

Our twin boys, now age 20, were on their own—Christopher was living in Waco, Texas, working at Magnolia Market, and Matthew was working full time at a local grocery store in Houston and was living with friends. We were starting to experience the freedom of "empty nesting" after being married 33 years and were making plans to travel and pursue other interests without children. Remembering our fun times together in our 20's before raising our kids, we were planning some vacations and visiting friends like we did years before. We were also "cruisers" in our earlier years, starting our honeymoon with a Disney cruise. Over the years, we'd even taken the boys with us on two cruises. In the time since they left the house, we had enjoyed two cruises by ourselves and were loving our freedom.

My cousin Tod McCoy (my aunt's son on my father's side) had left me a couple of phone messages over the holidays in late 2020. We had gotten along when we were growing up, and he visited us in Tucson when the boys were in elementary school. He had recently moved to Montana to be with his future wife, Nikki, so I thought he wanted to do the regular holiday catch-up phone call. On January 1, 2021, when my husband and I were both home with mild cases of Covid, I sat down on our living room couch and decided to return his call while Chris was cooking dinner.

There are always one or two people in every family that have the interest and energy to work on family genealogy. Tod was that person on my Dad's side. After catching up on family news, Tod asked if I had ever been interested in doing a DNA test like 23andMe. I remember thinking, "that's an odd, random, and kind of personal question," but I also remember having a nagging feeling—a red flag—that he could have a bigger reason for asking me. The story that unfolded during that conversation would create the biggest pivot I could have ever imagined.

Tod explained that he had been contacted recently through 23andMe by someone who claimed to be a cousin living in Nashville. The person mentioned that he had been the result of a donation of sperm or an embryo. Tod then asked me if that might ring a bell with what we did in our fertility journey?

The world stopped turning for a few seconds as my mind spun faster than the rotation of the earth. I felt the blood drain out of my face. I got Chris' attention—waving for him to come back to the couch. I put the phone on speaker and told Tod that sperm donation and embryo donation were very different. Seeing that many of my relatives spent a lot of time in Tennessee while I was growing up, sperm donation could have potentially been done by several people. But embryo donation—well, that's another thing.

Tod continued to tell us about the contact he had with the person on 23andMe, and later sent us the actual email conversation.

On December 17, 2020, Tod received a message through 23andMe from Thomas Monroe IV.

> *Hi I'm Thomas. I was adopted into a family from a sperm donor. My adoptive parents didn't know the male and female (I was a frozen embryo given to my adoptive mom) and I just thought it would be cool to try and connect with them.*

Tod wrote Thomas back that same day:

> *Hi Thomas: very nice to meet you! I'm intrigued by your story—the science says that you're my first cousin by way of one of my aunts or uncles, but honestly the dates of their births don't hold up. If alive today, they'd all be anywhere from 83-101 years old! I'm wondering if it's a younger member of the family and 23andMe just got the relationship wrong. I'd love to help, so please let me know if there's anything I can do. (One thing that*

would help is if you are connected to other people who might be connected to me. That could help narrow it down.)

Cheers,
Tod

Answer from Thomas (12/17/20)
Hey Tod. That is really interesting. I just got started on the app not too long ago so I will do my best to find out.

It was during that time from Dec. 17 through the end of 2020 that Tod reached out to me asking for the holiday phone call.

Tod couldn't remember exactly what procedure we had gone through to have the twins, but he knew it was some sort of infertility treatment. As Tod investigated the situation, he learned that the genetic relationships revealed through 23andMe claimed that he was a direct cousin. Tod's first thought was "Whoops! Someone wasn't careful!!" But, Thomas said he was the result of a frozen embryo donation. So, Tod looked into family history and compared dates of birth, at his aunts and uncles, and wondered who the donor(s) might be. But none of them fit the profile—neither by age nor personality. It wouldn't have been HIS father, as the DNA results would have said so. The closest candidate would have been MY father, but he died long before Thomas was born, and if he DID donate, the sample would have been sitting around for quite a number of years.

He was stumped. Maybe 23andMe got the relationship wrong and the donor was NOT an uncle?

The donor certainly wasn't Tod. It could have been his brother, Tim, but the DNA results would have been more exact. My brother Barry? Don't think so. No one on Tod's side of the family seemed like a viable candidate, but the men on my side of the family COULD have been candidates.

We were a longshot—and Thomas did mention something about embryos. As we explained a synopsis of our story to Tod, the reality of the story came into view for all of us. We all three took deep breaths, realizing the gravity of what we were learning and the possible repercussions of that information.

Chris and I didn't have to talk about the next steps, because we had talked about it frequently over the years. Being true to what we had said many times, we asked Tod to clarify the embryo donation versus sperm donation. If embryo donation was the true situation, we gave Tod permission to give him my email address.

We realized the significance of what was potentially being revealed. I was cautious and didn't want to raise any false hopes. I needed more information before confirming what I thought.

In the meantime, we found 18-year-old Thomas C. Monroe on Facebook. He showed up immediately on my search, with a little icon photo of a good looking young man with glasses and a solid jawline. Tears bubbled as I looked at his picture. The resemblance to my boys, and to my brother, was remarkable. No, it was impossible. I showed the picture to Chris and exclaimed, *"THIS HAS TO BE OUR KID!"*

After talking with me, Tod responded to Thomas.

January 2, 2021, from Tod to Thomas:
Hi Thomas -- Hope you're well and had a happy new year. I know of someone in the family who donated, but need a little more information: Do you know what facility that you as a frozen embryo came from?

Response from Thomas:
Not off the top of my head. Let me ask my dad

Response from Tod:
As long as you're asking, you might check to see whether you were a donated sperm or a donated embryo -- they're two entirely different things, and it would help narrow things down. (You mentioned both in your original message.)

From Thomas to Tod:
I was from an embryo but my dad isn't sure if I'm from a donor or a couple.

Response from Tod:
Do you know what facility it was from?
Thomas, you should write to my cousin Brooke who will have more information about your situation. Please keep in mind that this is a pretty heavy thing, to find out who your biological parents are, and it's going to change people's lives. If this is something you really want to know more about, then you should write to her. I think we know who your parents are, but Brooke wants more information before we can say anything definitive because there are still too many variables. So, it will require you to find out more information first -- if you can find out what facility you came from, that will seriously narrow things down. If you want to proceed, then write to Brooke at xxxxxxxxxx@gmail.com.
I wish you all the best!
Tod

Thomas:
Thanks Tod! I really appreciate the help and I will find out about the facility.

First email from Thomas to Brooke on Jan 2, 2021:
Hello, my name is Thomas. I got 23andme a couple months ago and started talking to Tod McCoy. He said that I should contact you about any info about my biological family. All I know is that my adoptive parents said that I was an embryo that was donated. If this is something you would like to talk about, please reply to this email.

At this point, the truth of the situation was staring right at us. Cautiously, I wrote him back later that day. Either this could be our biological child, or it could be a big misunderstanding. I wanted to be kind, not maternal, and factual. Inside I was feeling excited, nervous, and even a bit numb. The situation felt unreal.

My response, Jan 2:
Hi Thomas,

Good to hear from you. The info you sent Tod mentioned both donated sperm and a donated embryo...do you know which one it is? Did your parents adopt an embryo (egg + sperm) and then your mom gave birth after it was implanted? I know that's some technical info but it makes a difference in the story. Once I know more I might have more info.

Also wondering if your parents are ok with you seeking out this info?

Thanks and God bless,
Brooke Martin

I was hoping that this 18-year-old would check his email over the weekend and would answer me in the next few days. But within an hour, I received an answer.

Sat Jan 2, 9:22 PM from Thomas:
It was an embryo that my mom then gave birth to me and my siblings (I'm a triplet) and yes my dad is perfectly ok with it. He's actually the one who bought me the test.

I read the email once, twice, and again. I read it out loud to Chris. "Does that say triplets? What does that mean...3 children are ours? Three babies?" I just couldn't take in this incredible information. After all these years, learning within the past 24 hours that there could be THREE? So many variables, so many questions. We took a deep breath and kept asking, clarifying, praying.

I was terrified.

Sat., Jan. 2 9:27 PM
From Brooke

Oh my...are the triplets all biologically 100% siblings?
I held my breath for the answer.

9:32 PM
Yea. The doctors told my parents that they put in 2 embryos but they actually put in 3, and then my mom gave birth to us. C-section though but still.

All these years, I worried and prayed and asked for a sign so that my curiosity and selfish need to know could be satisfied. And God had been doing THIS all along! Breaking through the fog, feelings of joy and shock covered me. I realized that nothing I could have imagined happening to those embryos would have resulted in the miracle that I was experiencing. I was amazed by God's sovereignty at that moment. It turned out that the fate of those babies had nothing to do with God satisfying any of my desperate need to know—but everything to do with HIS plan for those precious children and their family.

We always joked that if there were other kids out there, they would probably be all boys since there are more boys in our families than girls. But what if I had a daughter? I'd never even considered it. Until now.

More emails continued into the night.

9:43 PM from Brooke
Wow Thomas....God bless your mom and dad! Are your siblings all boys?

We may need to talk more...it's a possibility that those embryos were mine/my husbands. We have twin boys that are 20 now, and we donated the extra embryos in hopes that they would find a good family. I don't want to jump to conclusions, but we are definitely open to finding out. We are still married and respect the decision that your mom and dad made 18 years ago. We don't want any information to affect your relationship with your parents.

Please talk to your parents and see what steps you all (and your siblings?) want to take next. If you want to exchange pics I'm fine with that too.

Also we live in Texas now...

God bless you!
Brooke Martin

13 minutes later....at 9:56 PM from Thomas:
We are actually 2 boys and a girl! And my dad is all open for it and knows it won't affect our relationship. My dad was adopted as well and he actually found his biological family which gave me the idea to get a test. We are 18 now and we live in Tennessee. I will text my siblings and see if I can send pictures.

My eyes now filled with tears again—two boys and a girl. A daughter! What in the world was happening?

Another email from Thomas 2 minutes later:
I also forgot to mention that in the 23andme predicted family tree, there is a predicted uncle for me by the name of B Martin who has almost the same genetic stuff as mine.

The identification of B Martin as an uncle solidified the story in our eyes. That would be Chris' brother Bret Martin, whose genetic information was also on 23andMe.

By this time, Chris had become more concerned about the expectations and interactions with Thomas' parents. He wanted to make it clear that we are not their parents and that we didn't want to cross any boundaries or put ourselves into parental roles. We tried to center our thoughts and wanted to ask appropriate questions while showing Thomas that we were thrilled to hear all the news.

10:17 PM From me with pics included:
Yes that B Martin is in Charlotte, NC! We know that he has

had his DNA done but we have not. Omigosh! I'm just stunned. Here are some pictures...can tell you more details soon. I think I found you on Facebook so I will send you a friend request…

11 minutes later, at 10:28 PM from Thomas:
Ok so Christopher has my sister's chin, which none of us have, and Matthew has the same kind of smile and eyes as my brother. I showed it to my dad and he agreed with me. I'm absolutely shook. My brother is putting a little bit more thought into it but my sister is on board. And I can update you on that tomorrow as well.

His sister is on board? She wanted to talk to me? I wondered if I could get to meet her—and the boys? I tried to control my excitement, but my mind just couldn't let go of the incredible facts that I had just learned.

10:51 PM from me to Thomas
Thomas, we are pretty "shook" too! But honestly very happy and blessed! We always said if anyone ever found us we would welcome them and KNOW we did the right thing!

I look forward to learning more about you. I will tell my boys when the time is right...they know the story and that there is a possibility that you were out there.
Sleep well!

Sleep? What sleep? The emails continued into the night that Saturday night.

10:52 PM from Thomas
I will let my siblings know if they want to know more. I'm really looking forward to talking and learning more about you guys!

I had a million things to ask but didn't even know where to

start. I was so anxious to see pictures of everyone—especially the girl. I didn't even know her name yet!

10:57 PM from Brooke
Tell your sister I look forward to seeing pics of her...I only had the 2 boys so always wondered what a girl would look like/be like!

11:46 PM from Brooke
I am still wide awake...wondering if any of you are musical or play sports? Matthew was a football player at his 6A high school and was starting varsity center his senior year. He played football at a D3 college for a year but came home during Covid and decided to change schools. He is studying to be a process engineer for the oil/gas industry.

Christopher is an incredibly gifted musician...played gigs around town in high school and was known for his music in high school and church. He is the music director at a church in Waco and works at Magnolia Farms (the Chip and Joanna Gaines place). Both sports and music/art run in the genes...will tell you more soon!

11:57 PM from Thomas
I actually wrestle for my school. Sadly we're in Nashville and Tennessee is taking extra precautions due to Covid and has not announced a schedule. My sister is a talented musician, who mainly sings but plays some guitar. She sometimes sings for our church, Christ Presbyterian Church. My brother is a gamer but he is very talented with his job at a pizzeria.

His brother works at a pizzeria? The sister is a singer and plays guitar? At this point the similarities between the triplets and my twins and us rendered the situation more plausible to me. I don't believe in coincidences, so I know that God had given all of these kids certain giftings that couldn't be denied.

As I looked through Thomas' Facebook posts, I saw pictures of him in high school and others who I assumed were his siblings. It was easy to overload on information because there were so many pictures. Within a few minutes, I discovered the one upsetting event that has happened in this whole story: Thomas had lost his mother, Becky Monroe, only a year before. She was the woman that probably bore my biological children, and I wouldn't get to meet her. It hit me hard; my thoughts now went to their father, the triplets, and all they had been through. They had lived an entire life with all of the ups and downs, and now this tragedy. I strangely wished I could have been there for them, that I somehow knew them and wanted to protect them from heartaches.

I only went to sleep because I didn't want to keep Thomas up all night, but any sleep I had was filled with thoughts of all of the questions I needed to ask the triplets. I felt so grateful that Thomas had decided to reach out to us; but I also was worried that the magnitude of the situation might be too much for an 18-year-old to handle.

> Sunday, January 3, 2021 - Shock
> From Brooke to Thomas, 8:30 AM:
> *I hope you are doing ok…I really thought about and prayed for all 3 of you and your dad last night. I know this is heavy information and I want it to be a positive experience for all of us!*
>
> 8:32 AM from Thomas
> *Thank you. And I pray that it wasn't hard on you guys either. I mean finding out that those embryos were put to good use must have been a great but shocking feeling.*

Wow! He seemed like such a nice young man. That he asked how we were doing was very meaningful to me, and I felt comfort that we were all going through the similar shock of learning about each other.

8:49 AM from Brooke
Yes exactly and we feel so blessed to know! How would you like to move forward? We are leaving it up to you, ok?

I saw on your Facebook that you may have lost your mom last year. That makes me so sad because I would have loved to know her. 😢

I may be jumping the gun to assume that this is all accurate, and we do want to do DNA testing to make sure. But with the finding of relatives on both sides, and the rarity of adoptive embryos, I feel pretty sure about it.

You do have some bio relatives still in Tennessee. I was born and raised in Cookeville, and we lived in Sparta until 2002.

Just think about it and ask whatever you want to know, ok? We would really like to have a conversation with your dad at some point if possible.

Ok....let me know what info you want to start with. We are around today...

Funny thing you said your brother works in a pizzeria...well my husband was a Pizza Hut manager/district manager for 20 years! 😊

9:20 AM from Thomas, with pictures:
This is my sister Lauren. She is technically the oldest out of the three of us. I will try to send a video of her singing because she actually sounds a lot like Christopher but in a higher pitch.

A picture of my biological daughter. I didn't have any expectations at all. But my first reaction was that she was beautiful and unique, and she looked a lot like Christopher. *And she sang?* I wanted to know everything about all three of the Monroe kids, but knowing about Lauren was magical.

I suddenly had a reaction that I wasn't expecting. I longed to learn what they were like as babies, as toddlers and as young teenagers. I felt like my curiosity was selfish, and I knew I would never get an answer. I had never gotten to put bows in a little girl's hair, or have tea parties with a daughter. I never longed or wished for that when I was raising my boys, but now that I knew that I had a biological daughter, I started wondering. And I wanted to know more about her.

9:28 AM from Brooke
Wow, she is so beautiful! Three great-looking kids (ok adults, kinda lol).

You are all having to go to school and graduate remotely? How annoying!

So, tell Lauren that my mother was an artist and my dad was a musician.

Thomas let me know that he was at work the rest of the day but would email me as soon as he could. I took advantage of that, as the questions in my head were taking over my sanity by Sunday. It had been just 48 hours since we found out about the triplets, and just to do anything normal, like housework, was hampered by a fog of emotions that day. On top of that, we were still testing positive for Covid, and although neither one of us were very sick, we were physically and emotionally exhausted.

We realized at this point that we would have to tell our boys that they now had three more 100% biological siblings, including a sister. My precious boys that God chose for us…would they be upset? Would they be jealous? What would this situation look like in the future?

Monday, Jan. 4, 7:39 AM from Brooke:
Thomas,

I wanted to let you know that I haven't told my boys about you at this point. I want to wait until you are ok with it and until we can connect with your dad. However, I would love to…I think they would be joyful too.

We are planning on doing a DNA test soon to make sure, as well.

How are you feeling about it?

7:53 AM from Thomas
I think that is a great idea. I'll shoot my dad a text right now so I don't forget.

Lauren was asking me if I had any more info from last night when I got home! She is invested in it as well.

Thomas seemed so easy going about this news. He was transparent and honest through these first conversations, and I could tell he was well-spoken and mature. My hopes in hearing from Lauren kept me from sleeping that Sunday night. I didn't know what to expect or how to respond to a daughter.

Monday, Jan 4, 11:05 AM. First Email from Lauren:
Hi Mrs. Martin!

I just wanted to shoot you an email introducing myself and saying hi. When I was told the possible news about all of this, I was overwhelmed and excited all at once. I don't know a whole lot of information about it all considering Thomas has been the one you've been talking to.

If you'd like to email me more about everything I would love that, but if not I'd totally understand. All of this is still pretty new.

Thanks!

Lauren

Oh God. This is real!

My biological daughter was emailing me. Should I even call her a daughter? The train of thoughts in my head were countless. She had a beautiful mom I'm sure she missed. I felt like I needed to walk on eggshells at that point with all of the kids. She called me Mrs. Martin in the email. But what else could she call me? Brooke? Biomom? No, that had the word "mom" and wasn't appropriate. I guess Mrs. Martin was the best choice at this point. But I didn't want her to think it needed to be that formal.

My response 11:28 AM:
Oh Lauren! How exciting to hear from you! Yes, it has been a whirlwind, hasn't it?

As I told Thomas, I'm going to leave the door open and you can ask whatever you want. My husband and I knew that a time like this might come, but to hear triplets is amazing.

I am also writing your dad an email because I want him to be OK with all this. We have no expectation of having a parental relationship with any of you, but we are willing to learn more about each other and see what happens.

Your brother sent me pictures and you're so beautiful! As he also told you, we have a lot of music in our family so would love to talk to you about that.

I'm getting ready to run some errands so will email more this afternoon. But feel free to ask me anything. We are just so happy

*and really praising God that the three of you are doing well.
:-)*

Lauren's Response: 11:40 AM
Of course! My dad went through a similar situation with his biological family I think about 4 years ago. As he'll probably tell you, he's giving each of us the opportunity to choose what we want out of this.

As for the music aspect, it's so relieving to hear that! I would love to talk more about that and other things like, are you guys good at art?

I'm pretty good at art, and my mom was too but she'd always wondered who I got it from.

Send me an email back whenever is convenient for you.

Are we good at art? I laughed out loud. My mom was an art professor and my father was a music professor, so apparently Lauren and I had a lot to talk about! My joy was immeasurable.

My response 12:45 PM
Wow that's a loaded question and one I'm pleased to answer!

My mother was actually an art professor at Tennessee Tech University, and my dad was a musician. My mom passed away 6 years ago but was fairly well respected in the area. Her name was Sally Crain-Jager and she was a painter. You can Google her and find info about her, too.

My father died in 1994. He played the French horn in the Nashville Symphony for many years when I was growing up. My brother is also an incredibly talented artist and has done original pencil work for Marvel and DC comics' story boards. Once we feel like we can tell our kids about you, I will be able to give you more information about my son who is a musician. I did find your Facebook page and we listened to your beautiful voice. You favor our musician son in your looks and your voice! This is incredible.

You can find me on Facebook as Brooke Elise Martin. A flowery background and a pic of me. :-)

12:50 PM Response from Lauren:
That's incredible! So weird too because I actually played French horn through middle and high-school up until senior year. It's so relieving to find out where I get my talents from! Is there anything you'd like to know??

What? She played *French Horn?* How is that even possible… how many teenage girls play the French horn? At this point in the communication, some of our amazement started turning into humor. The similarities between the Monroe kids and my boys, and between the triplets and other biological relatives were so incredible.

From there, Lauren and I exchanged phone numbers and started communicating via text.

Our next task was emailing their father, Trey Monroe. We decided to be totally transparent and to accept anything he might say. Since we found out he'd lost his wife, we were worried that our presence in his life might cause more stress. So, I wrote a very carefully worded email to the man who was probably the birth father of our biological children.

First Email to Trey Monroe: Monday, Jan 4, 6:24 PM
Good afternoon!

Well... what a weekend! I was so blessed to be able to email your amazing son, Thomas, and compare notes on the potential match of donated embryos. My husband and I want to first reach out to you and make sure that you are OK with all this. We have known this could've been coming for 20 years, so we are feeling very blessed and joyful to hear about all three of the kids.

We want you to know that we are thankful for the risk that you and your precious wife took to bring life into the world. It means the world to us because now we know we made the right decision to donate... which was made very prayerfully and carefully 18 years ago. As Thomas may have told you, I have 20-year-old twin boys and they know the story as well, but we have not told them yet about your kids until we talk to you.

I have had tears many times this weekend as I have seen pictures of Thomas, Peter and Lauren, and know they've had a good life. I was very saddened to see that you lost your wife fairly recently, and I sure would have loved having the opportunity to thank her as well.

We are going to leave any "moving forward" in this to you and your kids. We have no intention or need of being a parent figure to any of them, but I appreciate knowing about them and answering any questions that they might have. Anything in addition would be icing on the cake for us.

We do plan on having a DNA test ourselves, but for the information that Thomas has provided from both sides of our family, it seems pretty apparent that they are our biological children. Although we live in Texas now, there are still some relatives in Tennessee. Both my parents' and my husband's parents have already passed away, but there are many cousins throughout Oklahoma, Tennessee, and North Carolina.

I'll look forward to hearing from you! Would be glad to have a phone call or a FaceTime conversation as well.

Many blessings,
Brooke and Chris Martin

What would we have felt like if we had been the ones to raise the triplets? There were many emotions, including anger, jealousy and denial among others. I wanted so badly for the connection to go well. It was something I had wondered about for 20 years. I was preparing myself for any response based on the heaviness of the situation.

I could have never imagined the response that we received less than 30 minutes later.

Hey guys, Trey Monroe here. Thank you for your kind email. I need to start by thanking you both for the gift of your children. My wife found meaning for her life and calling in Christ in being their mom. Being their father has been the adventure of my life. So from the depths of our hearts, thank you.

Becky and I shared their beginnings story when they were 12, I think. We were and are pleased for them to contact you guys, but support and honestly suggest that you take things slowly. I have my own reunification story which has been honestly wonderful, but the sheer amount of feelings I dealt with then was, well, interesting!

Thomas and Lauren are so excited, they share the photos of you guys and their must be brothers and are fairly buzzing! Thomas came in BIG eyed when you shared the number of stored embryos with him! Peter is feeling unsettled. He feels things deeply and is processing what this all means. I have shared with him that it is his life and his choices and that I will support him. I told him I understood any loyalty concerns he might have, but that our family could only be enhanced by this development.

I think his sibs are a little dismayed at his reaction but want to support him. Peter is deep and ponders things, no doubt like one of you or your family, and he is working things out. He was so close to his mom, I wonder if he feels unsettled by the news. I can share my perspective in a couple of days, and see if that helps him.

He did laugh when I asked to send some photos with him in them, the laughing came when I told him your sons were about to be surprised and out voted!.

All the kids are great. Becky and I loved each other deeply and them as much. We raised them in a Bible believing church, prayed for them, worried over them, and spanked them when they needed it. No doubt like you did. I believe we will all come through this interesting and blessed process the better for it.

I appreciate your intentions and know I will support the wellbeing of your family as well. I imagine we will be in touch again. God bless you four.

Trey

I cried—and still cry—when I read his email. God placed those embryos in the exact family that we prayed for. A woman who is a Christ-follower and wanted to be a mother. A couple who desperately wanted to have a family together. And a father who is so gracious.

I've tried to find the words to describe the feelings I had when I received that e-mail from Trey. Many of the emotions throughout our story are hard to explain because they've been so unexpected. Joy would cover it, although disbelief would too. All the things that we prayed for our embryos had just been proven true. I think I was just waiting for "the other shoe to drop," as they say. Something negative, something that would block the way to knowing more. I even searched, but there was nothing in that e-mail to indicate anything but understanding and love covering our entire story.

As human beings, we seem to expect the negative and not the positive. Through my experience, I learned that God really does want to bless us. He has to do it in his own way because he sees the big picture. The blessings I felt after reading that e-mail were overwhelming…nearly traumatic. Almost too good to be true. But it WAS true!

Answer from Brooke:
Trey,

We are just so thankful that all of our prayers seem to have been answered! We prayed for the Christian family that would raise the kids just like you did, including the spanking when needed! It must have been a riot with triplets!

We will take your advice to heart and work on building a relationship with each child at their speed. I told Thomas and Lauren that just knowing that they are OK is enough, anything else is icing on the cake. There are many parents who never would have revealed the origin of their conception, so the fact that you did that shows us what great, loving parents that you are. You can imagine the situations that could have happened and ran through our heads over the last 20 years. And again, I sure wish that I could've met your wife and thanked her in person as well. What an amazing woman!

We are an open book, so we will answer any questions. We plan on talking to our boys in a little while and then we'll see what happens.

Talk to you soon,
Brooke Martin

Telling our boys

The next phone call that Monday night was with our boys. Our "twinkies" that we prayed for and loved so much. I did not want this to affect their vision of me, of their dad, or of our tight-knit nuclear family. We scheduled a Facetime call and let them know it was important. We were both still Covid positive, so a virtual meeting was necessary.

They were both very curious, as you can imagine, on why we were having this family meeting. I've tried to recall exactly what we said, but I believe I started out with *"remember the story of those frozen embryos and how there could be other kids out there?"* I saw their eyes get big. *"Yes, it actually happened."*

"WHAT," they both said. *"Are you serious?"*

"Yes", I answered. *"We got a call last week. They found cousin Tod on 23andMe. You have other siblings."* One of the boys asked, *"Plural? We have more than one other sibling?"* Yes I said—actually three and they are triplets. They both broke into nervous laughter at that point, with their hands on their foreheads, shaking their heads. They were all smiles, and I couldn't have been happier and more relieved that they were smiling at that point.

Then I dropped the bomb. *"Guess what? One of them is a girl! You have a sister."*

As the conversation continued, we told them that we found Thomas's picture on Facebook. Since they were on their cell phones for the Facetime call, they simultaneously went there and found his profile. The looks on their faces told us: they knew that he was their brother. There was no doubt in their minds.

I told them that Thomas and Lauren had given their permission to find them on social media. Within a couple hours of our call, they connected with them and started communicating.

Later, I revisited that moment with each of the boys, and they both told me that since we had talked about the possibility over the years, it wasn't a completely new idea to them. They were curious about the other kids and wanted to know more. Matthew told me that he "wanted to see if they were good people," and Christopher wanted to be a good influence and for there to be a family relationship.

Within two days of telling my precious boys, Christopher found a video on Facebook of Lauren singing several years earlier and recorded another video of himself singing to her audio. He recorded the video in his car and sent it to me without any warning. It was on Wednesday night, two days after I told the boys about their triplet siblings. I was standing in the kitchen when I got the video of voices blending like angels. It was unbelievable and still gives me chills when I listen to it. My eyes filled with tears, my legs were weak, and my head went down on the kitchen table. I found myself weeping. My son and my daughter—singing together. Thank you, God.

One of the most surprising parts of the kids all knowing about each other is that they started communicating without my knowledge. As the mom, you think that you know everything that happens with your kids. So, it was surprising when Matthew would tell me he texted Lauren or he saw on social media that Thomas was working out. I wanted to say, *"What do you mean you talk and you didn't tell me?"*

After telling our boys, we realized that our extended family also needed to know the news! Chris has four brothers and sisters and lots of cousins. We started making calls, and the joy and surprise in their voices were wonderful and such a relief. Everyone immediately agreed that they wanted to meet the new family members and support us in any way that they could. My side of the family was also happy and supportive. Overall, it was a whirlwind of joy being able to tell them that there were three more family members. I think everyone was in shock, but also very happy about the news.

Around this time, Chris and I decided to do a DNA test through 23andMe, just to verify. I was still so emotionally numb and processing all of the information. I told Chris that if other kids popped up on the DNA search to "bring it on" because the definition of family had radically changed. I really meant that, too!

Getting to know each other

The first time we had a phone call with Thomas, it was a little awkward. First of all, he was an 18-year-old boy. As I remember, there were many short questions-and-answers—especially about the Monroe siblings and their father. Thomas was very well-spoken and had a kind spirit. We kept stressing that there was no pressure to have a relationship with us, but he really seemed OK with it—which continues to surprise us and bless us to this day. We say he is "the one that started all this" for finding us on 23andMe. But we all agree that God has led this entire journey for all of us. Upon his request, we started putting together a document that covered any health concerns and health histories for them.

The first time we had a FaceTime call with Lauren, I was so nervous. A daughter—who looked like me—I wasn't sure what I would say! It was within the first few weeks of the discovery, and only 14 months after she'd lost her precious mom. She had friends surrounding her during the call to support her, so there were lots of giggles and talking from a roomful of 18-year-old girls. She was outgoing and sweet, and also well-spoken like her brother. She seemed excited to meet us and opened up about her mom during that first conversation. After we hung up, Chris said, "Wow she is kinda off the chain!" I responded. "No, honey, she is an 18-year-old girl with my outgoing personality!"

We were hoping that Peter would want to talk or FaceTime, but with Trey's help we realized that while Peter was accepting of the discovery of the biological connections, wasn't ready to jump into a getting-to-know-you relationship. We were ok with that and were just thankful to see pictures of him and learn about his personality. He was more soft-spoken and a hard worker, and he loved working at a Nashville pizza restaurant.

For the next few months of 2021, we emailed, had more phone, Facetime, and texting conversations. I also connected with the Monroes on Facebook and other social media platforms. The similar talents and interests between my boys and the Monroes were incredible. Thomas was very motivated by sports and excelled in team environments. He was already planning on being a history teacher and making college plans. His motivations, matter-of-fact attitude, and easygoing personality were much like our son Matthew's personality.

From the first conversation, Lauren asked if there were musical or art talents in the family. I just didn't know where to start! Lauren sent me pictures of drawings and paintings she had done, and I sent Lauren pictures of, and information about, her biological grandmother, the art professor. Chris' family also had musicians in it; his father played the stand-up bass in a Navy band, and there was a well-known German musician in his family in the 1800's.

When I told friends and colleagues about the discovery, it was very therapeutic. I was working as a marketer in the mental health field, and this type of news can be very traumatic. I have many therapist friends, and several of them asked me how I was holding up. I responded that I really didn't know. The human brain is not set up for this type of information, so it took a long time to find a place for it. My years working in mental health taught me that if you can tell the events from trauma (positive or negative) from beginning to end without skipping around, it can help your brain put things in place and have a positive outcome.

So, I started telling the story. And I loved the joy that it brought to others.

In one instance, I was at a lunch event with a table full of colleagues. Someone had heard my story and encouraged me to tell the group. When I got to the part about finding out that we had triplet biological children, I looked at one of my male colleagues, and he had happy tears running down his face. He and his wife had gone through fertility issues and connected with my situation. Since then, whenever I recount our story, I always ask the listener if they're familiar with IVF. If so, I warn them that our tale is very emotional, and I watch their reactions and their facial expressions as they hear what happened to us. The last thing I wanted to do is to have a negative impact on someone's life.

But as I quickly found out, our story is full of joy and hope. At the time the discovery happened, the world was shut down with Covid, and there wasn't much positive news. There were many people wondering where God was, and wondering "What happens next?" God reminded me that I wondered for 20 years what had happened to the embryos. Sometimes I asked God, then even bargained with Him on allowing me to find out:

Maybe if I did all the right things, then He would let me know?

Maybe I had messed up somehow, and I would never find out what happened to any of them?

Well, look what God did! For 20 years he was orchestrating HIS plan, not mine. Come to find out, God was not influenced by my childish begging and bargaining. To think I could have influenced God in His decisions to weave the pattern of life is just embarrassing. He did so much more than I could have ever imagined. From that moment, I have not been as anxious about my life, my job, my children's futures and my future.

> *"Do not be anxious about anything, but in every situation, by prayer and petition with thanksgiving present your requests to God. And the peace of God, which transcends all understanding, will guard your hearts and your minds in Christ Jesus."* Philippians 4:6-7

As a professional marketer, I recognized the positivity we could spread from our story. The potential was enormous. I was concerned that some might see our family as a circus act—an odd dysfunctional group that craved attention. But I knew that God wanted to use our story for good. I ran an idea by all eight people involved about starting a Facebook blog to document our story. My husband and Trey didn't seem to see what the big deal was, and I don't think any of the kids did either. But I did. Trey's input on the focus of our story solidified what our story should stand for, as he told me in an email:

> *Hey guys, great to hear from you. Thomas and Lauren are really enjoying getting to know you guys better and it is a joy to watch them.*

> *For Becky there were 2 main things to her part of the story. One was the sanctity of life. For us that was involved from the very start. The other important part for Becky is that the process allowed her to become a mother. And that was all she wanted.*

> *She would be excited at the idea of sharing the story with other people. She would just want to make sure she had a major role. Lol.*

> *I am happy and pleased to be supportive in any way that I can. I do not pretend to understand what God is up to with this*

multigenerational family shenanigans, but I am sure it is good.
Trey

I knew that this story was a gift to share with others. A friend of mine suggested *"Love Multiplied"* as a title, which felt right to me. So, in the spring of 2021, *Love Multiplied* was created on Facebook, and we started posting our story.

Our Love Multiplied

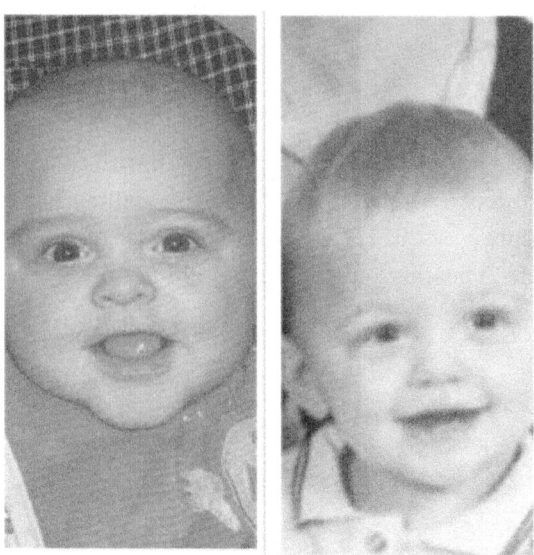

Peter Monroe (L) and Matthew Martin (R).

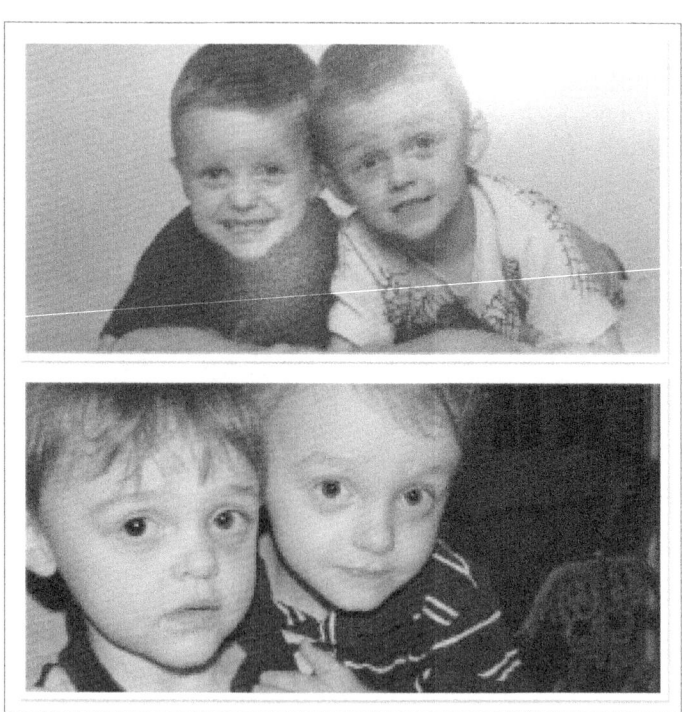

Top pic: Martin boys: Christopher and Matthew.
Bottom pic: Monroe boys: Peter and Thomas.

Lauren Monroe (L) and Christopher Martin (R).

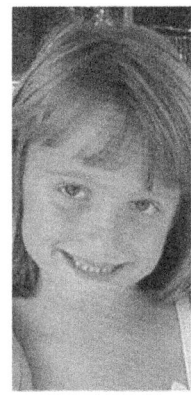
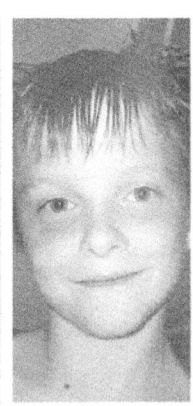

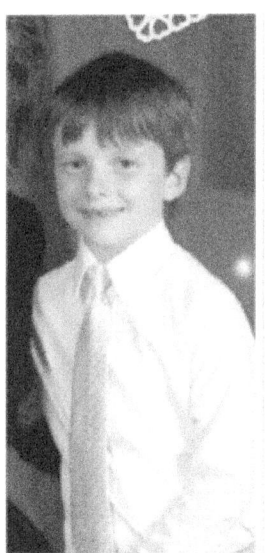
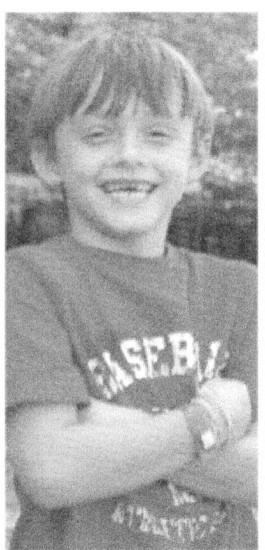

Christopher Martin (L) and Thomas Monroe (R).

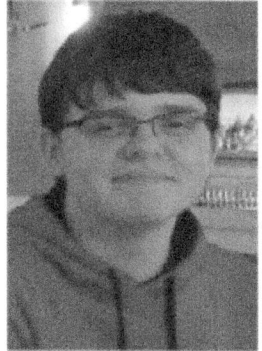 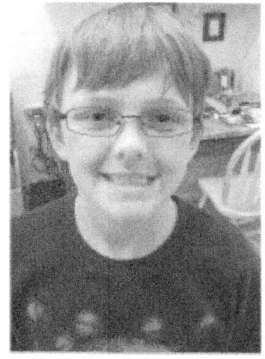

Peter Monroe (L) and Matthew Martin (R).

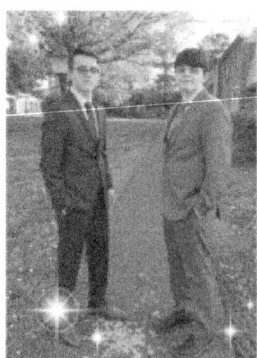 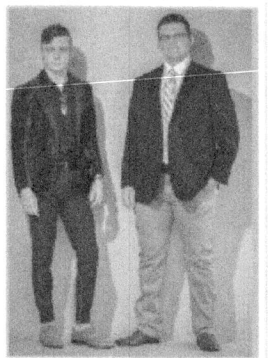

Monroe boys in left picture: Thomas and Peter.
Martin boys in right picture: Christopher and Matthew.

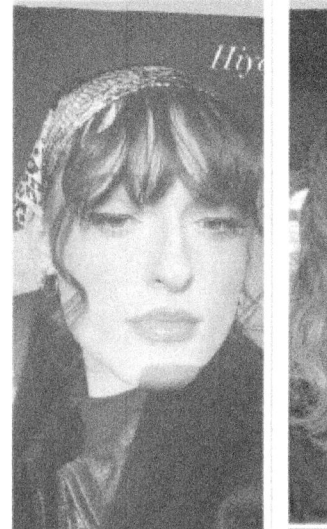
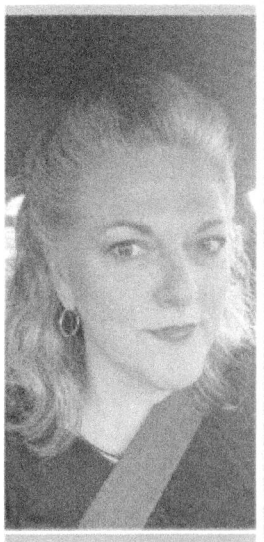

Both pictures: Lauren Monroe (L) and Brooke Martin (R).

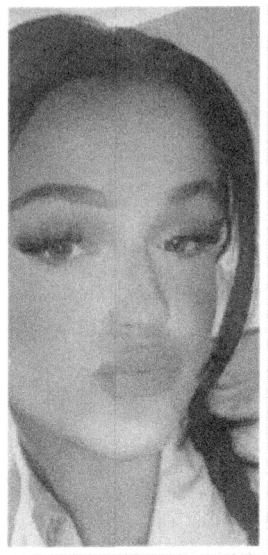
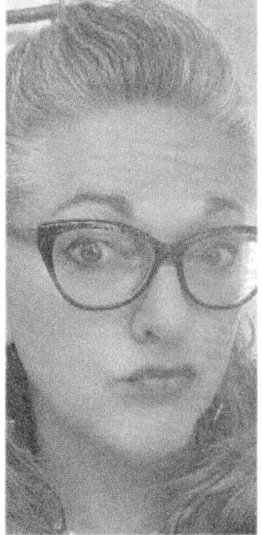

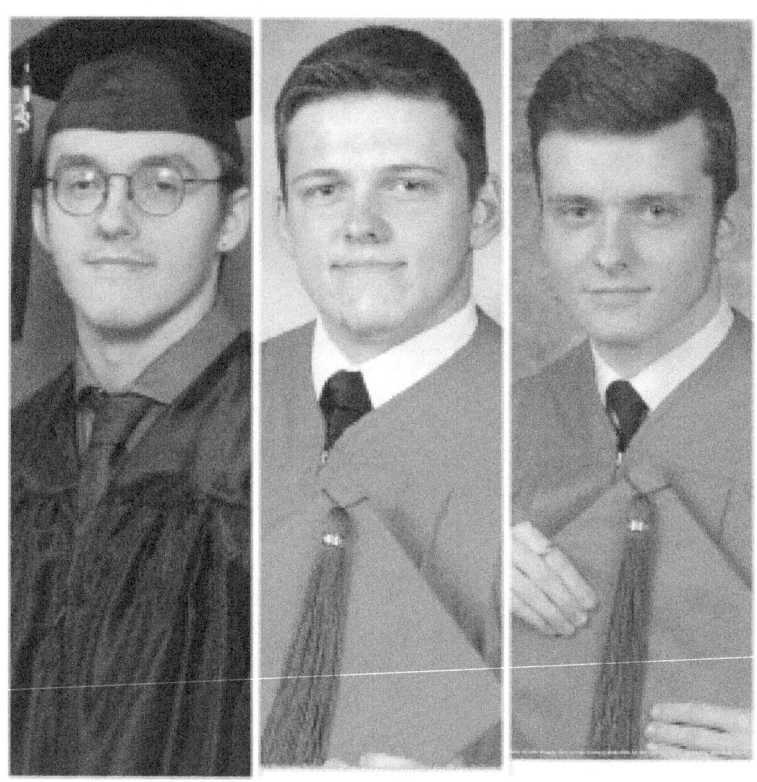

Thomas Monroe, Matthew Martin, and Christopher Martin.

All four boys: Top row: Thomas Monroe (L) and Peter Monroe (R).

Bottom row: Christopher Martin (L) and Matthew Martin (R).

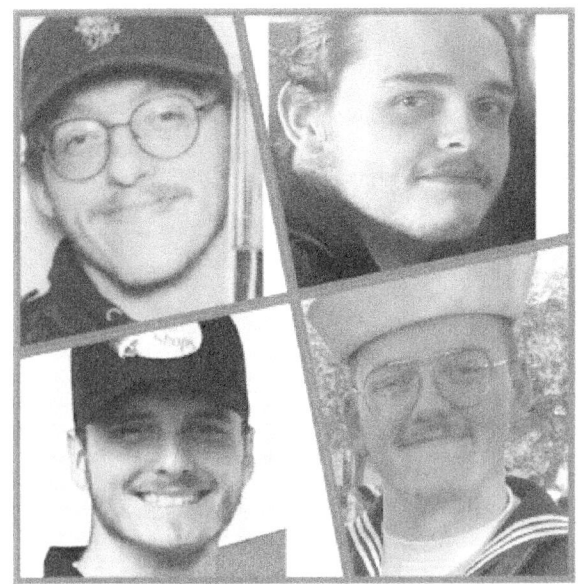

Thomas Monroe (L) and Christopher Martin (R).

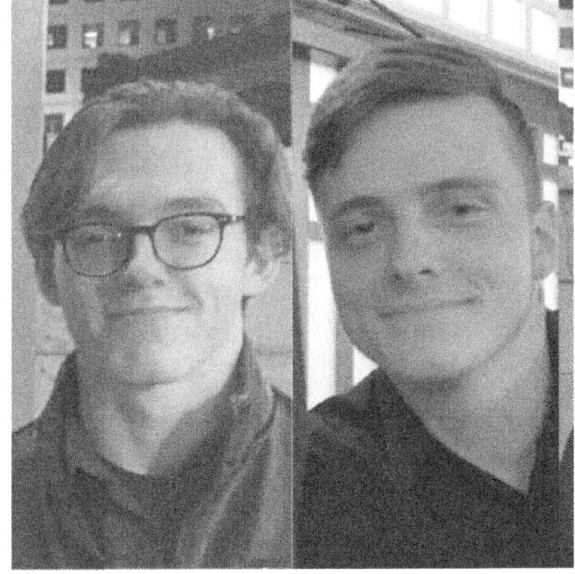

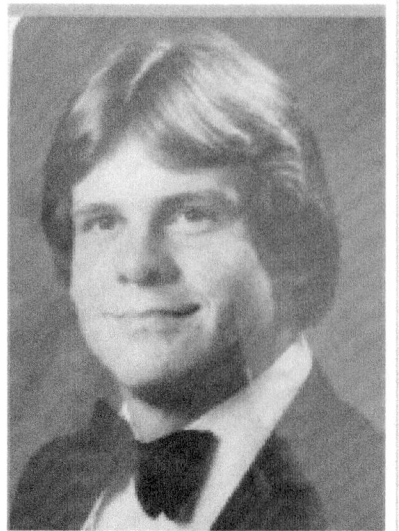
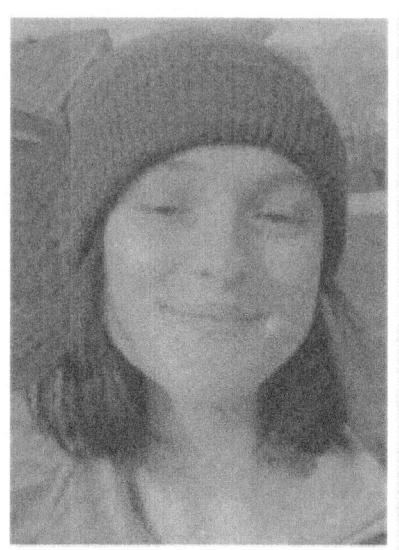

Chris Martin's high school senior picture (L). Lauren Monroe at the same age (R).

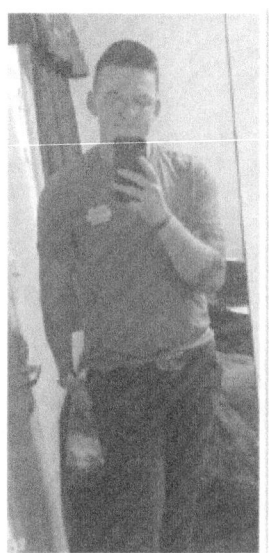
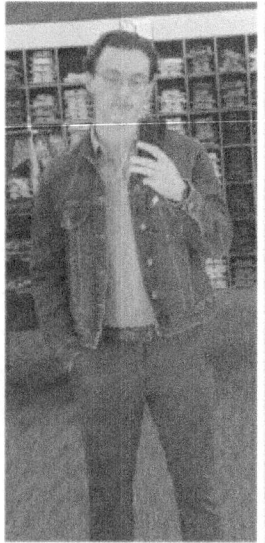

Matthew Martin (L). Thomas Monroe (R).

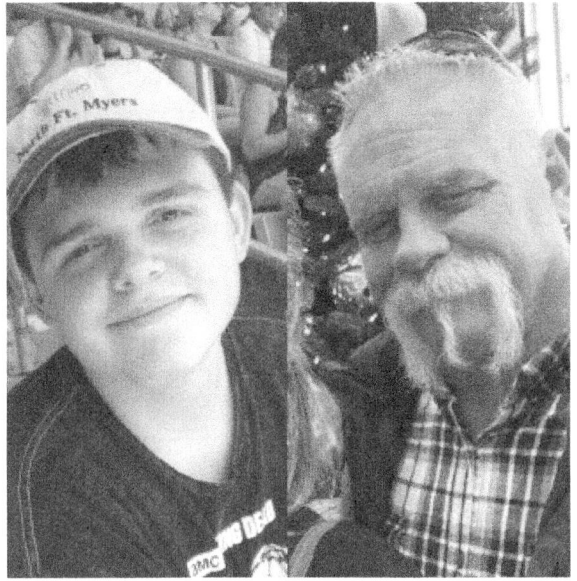

Peter Monroe and Chris Martin.

Part 3—The Monroes

The more I found out about the Monroes and their story, the more I realized the beautiful gift that was unfolding for all of us. There are many ways that our reunion could have gone wrong. So many stories about families finding each other have bad endings like expecting or even demanding money, inheritances, or special privileges. I have heard of families reuniting and then not getting along—even hating each other. During the discussions Chris and I had over the years about the "what ifs," those worries about the negative impact on our family and the potential newfound family weighed very heavily. The thought that everything would be good, a "rainbows and unicorns" ending, very rarely entered the realm of possibilities.

All of those possibilities kept creeping into my mind as I carefully navigated all the questions that I had about the Monroes. We had a joke: "Happy family is a Chinese dish." A truly balanced, normal family without any discord or drama just doesn't exist.

I couldn't even comprehend how this all could be impacting the three Monroe siblings, not to mention their father. The Monroe kids' devotion to their late mother Becky was so genuine and sweet, and the last thing I wanted to do was get in the way of any kind of relationships that they already had in their family. They had been through so much together with the fairly recent loss of their mom, and their emotions were raw. I was very nervous about asking for personal information or seeming to be too pushy. But both Trey and the kids gave me so much information that it was overwhelming.

Within the first few weeks after the initial emails, Trey was sending pictures of the Monroe triplets as babies and children. I saw pictures of my biological daughter as a toddler and as a developing teenager, and the similarities in the pictures between the Monroe kids and mine were breathtaking. Trey even sent me a link to an online portal of family videos. I could only watch them for short periods of time because they were so emotionally overwhelming.

There were videos of Lauren performing in choir, singing solos and playing guitar just like Christopher had done in high school. Videos of Thomas competing in wrestling matches with Becky cheering him on in the background. There were videos of the triplets acting goofy on family vacations. In every video or picture, I would catch glimpses of each child that had the same expression, grin, or mannerisms as my boys. It was an unreal experience, and still is!

As I learned more about them, I had to take breaks to let my mind absorb the information. My heart and brain had to process so much emotion, and although it was mostly joyful, other details emerged that solidified so much truth about God's love and sovereignty that had been proven in the Monroe family all those years.

On top of having access to watching the Monroe triplets grow up in pictures, the story that unfolded about Trey and Becky was deeply moving. The depth of the tapestry that had been woven together to create our stories convinced me beyond any doubt that God is the orchestrator of EVERYTHING. Not just in our family story but in my life and in a much bigger way. He had chosen this couple specifically for these children.

It's not that I had doubted God's sovereignty before, but the depth of truth was staggering. Navigating the world seemed to be simpler after this story unfolded. If God could do this, why am I worried about little things in life? Chris and I had our own story of a marriage restored, going through IVF, donating the embryos and raising our twins. Trey and Becky had also been through so much—even more than we had. My heart went out to them for what they had been through as well as the joy they experienced through the process.

The Monroes' journey

Rebecca Elizabeth Peter Monroe, "Becky," was a woman who had taken charge of her life. According to those who worked with her over the years, she was a memorable figure in the work of corporate healthcare human services in Nashville. Becky was almost six feet tall and had a commanding presence. Her ability to organize and conduct business led her to rise in the ranks at her company, which also required some travel.

After an earlier marriage in her late teens that lasted over a decade, she divorced but kept the townhome that the couple had bought. After a few years of being single, she met the love of her life, Trey Monroe, through dating ads in a local newspaper. Trey had worked as a photographer for many years, then went back to school to get his degree in psychology, then a post-graduate degree to be a psychologist. Trey's jovial personality and very dry wit, mixed with Becky's matter-of-fact attitude, balanced well.

Trey had a daughter from a previous marriage, Mary. After the couple wed, Becky took Mary in as her own. The three were happy, but Becky longed to expand their family. After three years of marriage with no pregnancy success and nearing 40 years of age, Becky realized that they might need to seek an infertility specialist.

They started their fertility journey in 2001, doing the same that we did in early 2000. After they checked into different options of fertility specialists, Becky and Trey went to Nashville Fertility Center. It is very possible that they were seeing the doctors there at the same time we were going through our own IVF process. I will never know, but I'm pretty sure that God had the dance figured out way before then and was watching it unfold with amusement.

According to Trey, the initial process was pretty easy, doing blood work, ultrasounds, and other tests on all of the important reproductive elements of both of them. After going through the required tests, the fertility clinic told them they could not help them.

Period.

They had gone in with high hopes. Nashville Fertility Center had a great reputation and had treated them with respect and professionalism. But they learned that Becky's eggs were prematurely aged and not viable, so they could not be used to create embryos for In Vitro Fertilization. According to Trey, Becky said something about knowing it was her problem. But Trey, with his dry and witty sense of humor, reminded her that he just had "three men in a boat." That made her laugh a little, as it was a reference to the TV show

Twin Peaks in which Sheriff Andy had a sperm count done and was initially told he had a low count; the doctor put it into terms he could understand, "three men in a boat." In truth, Trey's sperm count was between three men in a boat and a "whole darn town" as he said, but it was too low to have children. That helped ease the tension.

They expected an easy fix, so the "We are sorry we cannot help you" was a gut punch.

"You might want to look into adoption," the doctor offered. Becky was hopeful, but she later told her husband that she was a little worried that he would have favoritism for a biological child and it would cause parenting issues.

Another magical element of this story is that Trey himself was adopted as a baby and had a happy childhood. So, it seems that God had readied their hearts for the next steps. Becky would not be pregnant or give birth to a child if they adopted, something she very much wanted to experience, but they could raise and love the child together, and that would be wonderful.

So, they started looking into adoption. Since Becky was an organized and efficient person, she researched and found a social worker who would help with the process. It was someone she was familiar with from the local Jewish Community Center who provided adoption services. Becky took the reins of the project with Trey's full support. Eventually, a home study was done and interviews, together and apart, were completed. Psychological testing showed that Trey was mentally healthy and introverted, but did not like to be pushed too far. Becky's showed she was also mentally healthy but extroverted, and prone to self-doubt. The process went smoothly but a little slower than they wanted, according to Trey, until they were ready to get down to brass tacks, such as the gender and race of the potential baby.

When they met with the social worker, she presented the question, "How would you feel about adopting a child that is not white?" Becky and Trey hesitated for a moment, gave each other a quizzical look, and both said that was not an issue for them. Trey reminded the social worker that he had minored in African

American studies in college, and they would feel very comfortable in fostering a positive racial identity in a minority child.

"Would you consider a Mexican child?" the social worker asked. Again, the two exchanged glances and wondered why she was asking such a question. They said again, any race would be fine with them.

The social worker said she would get back to them soon with photos. It was about to happen! Although, they were confused as to how in the world you would choose a baby to adopt by viewing photos. That seemed strange and a little uncomfortable, but they were committed to the process.

Then they got a phone call.

It was the fertility clinic. *Again.*

At this point, Trey and Becky thought they were past help from the clinic, but they were intrigued enough to return the call and see what they might want.

"We may have an alternative for you," the doctor said. "Please come in, and let's discuss it."

Trey and Becky told the doctor that they were well on the way to adoption, but agreed to the consultation, thinking there had been some breakthrough in fertility treatments that might help them.

"What would you think about donor embryos?" Dr. Whitworth asked. She explained the process, how there were "left over" fertilized eggs that were unused from another couple's IVF treatments, and that the couple had instructed them to make the embryos available for other couples. We all put "left over" in quotes because we could not stomach labeling those embryos that way. Maybe using "extra" or "un-used" would be more appropriate.

The couple asked a few questions and then tried to wrap their heads around the concept, and quickly decided that it was completely acceptable. It was thought of as an adoption, just earlier in the process. But there was one problem: they could never afford it!

The baby adoption was quite expensive, and they assumed that the donor embryo situation would only cost more, so they laughed and said thanks, but they did not see a way they could pull it off.

Dr. Whitworth smiled and said, "It will cost you less than

$2,000 out of pocket, and your insurance will cover the rest." That was a game changer, and to this day Trey says it floored them. A typical adoption was going to cost $5,000 to $7,000 and did not involve doctors, so how could this price structure make sense? They were still unsure, but there it was. They were given some reading materials about the process, and they went home to ponder this new prospect.

Becky was excited because she would get to be pregnant and carry a child. That was a dream of hers that she thought had died. Trey was so happy for her, but it did not carry the same emotional weight for him. He did not care about the origin of their child; he just wanted them to have one. Her feelings on the matter were the heavier balance of the decision.

Since I also went through IVF, I know that preparing the woman's body for the process involved dozens of injections. It was still amazing to me that someone would go through that to carry babies that were not biologically hers. Becky's heart of acceptance had to be softened for many years—even a lifetime—to be open to that. She would have to prepare her body for a pregnancy and then go to the hospital to have the embryos inserted into her uterus, where they would potentially—and hopefully—thrive from there. Trey was concerned about the shots and worried about how painful they would be, but Becky was determined and motivated to go through the process no matter what it took.

Trey and Becky went back to the fertility clinic to begin, which involved getting the prescriptions for medications, syringes and everything needed to prepare her for the implantation of the embryos. They had focused on the process of implantation and until then had given little thought to the embryos and their origin.

The fertility clinic gave them a donor profile that we, the donor couple, had filled out about our health and social background. The thought that Becky and Trey looked at the exact document that we filled out less than a year before still gives me chills. We had donated the embryos in March of 2001. We estimate that they reviewed our information in January of 2002, ten months later.

When Trey and Becky reviewed the donor profile, nothing

unusual stood out, although every family has health concerns. There were some cancer, alcohol problems and other things in the donor family that started to concern them. As they discussed their feelings about it, Becky came up with a brilliant idea.

"Trey, let's fill this out for ourselves and see how they compare," she said. Trey loved the idea.

They created a comparison using Trey's adoptive family, since he had no information about his biological family. Among the characteristics he had to include were an abusive grandparent, glaucoma, and blindness, as well as normal genetic issues with Becky's family.

When they completed it, they compared the lists, and Trey concluded it was more than a match. "Honey, I think we're getting a bargain!" he declared. They laughed with relief, and that was the last worry they had about the donors of their little miracle. Trey recalls asking the doctor about the donor couple and remembers her smirking just a little, saying "Oh, they're a lot like you two." Becky and Trey were pleased with that answer and continued to move forward. We all appreciate that the clinicians at the fertility clinic saw that our families would be a great match, and we all know God had a great deal to do with it!

So just like us, they started with the injections. At first, Trey was able to inject most of the shots himself, but as things progressed, Becky was able to self-administer them into her thigh. It was a relief to Trey as he hated giving Becky the shots and was worried he would mess it up by hitting a nerve or who knows what. In time, Becky noticed the changes in her body as it prepared for the embryo implantation.

On the day of the implantation, Becky got cleaned and prepped, and they went into the hospital room where doctors prepared the equipment. Trey would also be involved. The doctors placed the end of the tube containing the embryos into her uterus, and Trey was given the official duty of depressing the plunger to push the two embryos into their future. Two? Yes, they were told, two. Each embryo had a 66% chance of successfully attaching to her uterus and starting the pregnancy. Given those odds, they would insert two embryos with the hope that at least one, and perhaps both, would be successful. Statistically, they would likely have only one baby, but there was a chance they could have twins. The prospect of this happening was a little frightening to both of them. One child seemed like a huge undertaking, and two was just a little silly, according to Trey. But they clung to the odds that they would be parents of a single child. Nice and normal. Trey pushed the syringe plunger in like a champ, and there were congratulations all around!

A few weeks later, Becky and Trey returned to the clinic for an ultrasound to see if any of the embryos had attached. The doctor was all smiles, but as she inspected the ultrasound, her smile vanished. Puzzled, she seemed to be counting under her breath. When she looked up at them, she seemed a little peeved when she asked, *"Why did you have three embryos implanted?"*

Three? Nobody said anything about three! There was silence in the room. Becky and Trey exchanged quick surprised glances before returning their focus to the doctor who was staring at the screen. *"There are three. Why did you implant three?"*

Trey shook his head. *"We haven't had much control in this whole process. We trusted you!"*

She looked back at the screen and announced: *"You're going to have triplets."*

Becky and Trey were dumbfounded. This was NOT part of the plan! Triplets? As in, three babies?

The doctor left the office to find out what had happened while Becky and Trey waited, stunned and silent. What the doctor found was that the process involved thawing three embryos, hoping for two that were A or A+ on the Gardner rating scale. The attending doctors, surprised that all three of the embryos were viable and high grade, found themselves in a quandary. They knew that our wishes as the donor couple were clear: to not harm or waste any of the embryos. And the doctors, like the Monroes, believed each embryo was a precious life. So, honoring our wishes, they implanted all three.

Who ultimately made the decision to implant all three embryos is still unclear. The doctor didn't tell Trey and Becky, their colleagues, or anyone so far as can be determined. Trey says that looking back, if the doctors would have told them or the physician who they had consulted, things would have only become clouded. Only God knew the outcome.

Fear

Friends suggested that Trey and Becky could sue the fertility clinic. They mulled it over, but concluded: How could they sue the doctors for making their dreams come true while honoring the wishes of the donors? Becky and Trey decided that in good conscience they couldn't do it. They dropped the idea.

But other ideas appeared. Fear set in, mostly financial. At their age, would they be able to raise three children? At once? It grew like poison ivy in their hearts.

The following is Trey's account of the days that followed:

The words not said during those first few weeks between my wonderful wife and I would fill volumes. Thankfully, we were created with rich emotional communication systems in our faces and bodies, and we used those to communicate the joy and fear and terror and confusion and hope and shock we shared. Becky called her best friend Cathy Matthews to share the news with her. Cathy loved Jesus, and Becky deeply appreciated and respected that. Becky laughed nervously as she spoke. And I recall being a bit dissociated myself.

My recollection and the story my wife endorsed (she did enjoy a good story, truth be told) was that I did not speak about the triplet pregnancy, nor much at all, for a period of weeks. It was too much to consider, more than I could hold at that time. Denial and shock, yes, that was it for me. So, I kind of shut down about it.

The fear got to us, especially to Becky. I was not angry, because I was as afraid as she was.

The most repeated commandment in Scripture is to not be afraid. There is a reason for this repetition.

Yet this situation frightened us to our bones.

Not being able to speak was not a story or a metaphor. Literally, I was struck dumb. Becky suffered from my silence until she broached the subject of selective abortion with me. Please do not abuse my honesty concerning our fear and desperation by judging my wife, my prize, my partner. That she spoke those words was indicative of how overwhelmed and hopeless she felt, no doubt exacerbated by the amazing pyrotechnics a pregnant mother of triplets experiences hormonally, and her experience of me being shut down and overwhelmed too.

"We can't do that. We just can't do that. We can give some of them or all of them up for adoption, but we cannot do that," Becky shook, sobbed, and melted into me. She repeated, "We cannot do that." She knew about my adoption and how that had been a blessing for me. Hope arose from her despair.

I knew what we could not do; we could not kill any life we had worked so hard to help create. As I said, we were terrified. But not as afraid as we soon would be.

It was Friday afternoon, just after five when Becky got home from work and looked pale and awful. "Trey, I'm bleeding. A lot." I held her as she called the doctor's office. She got a call back from our doctor who said it sounded like she was losing the pregnancy but to come Monday morning and we would see. The terror of losing our children was mingled with our utter shame over having discussed selective abortion.

We got on our knees and begged God to save our children. We confessed our fear and asked his forgiveness, then we got on the phone and called everyone we knew who had a knack for prayer. Some people do; they pray and things happen. All prayer is powerful, but some people evidently just do it better.

So that is how we spent our weekend. In shame and fear. Lovely.

We dreaded the Monday appointment, thinking God would judge us for our lack of faith and hard hearts. They did an ultrasound, and there were three fetuses, all implanted in her uterus as they should be. "I guess with three implanting there was more blood, so it was a false alarm," the doctor said. "Everything is fine and dandy!" In retrospect, God helped us get through our fear of having triplets by showing us something far worse—the fear of losing them. It worked. We never had any fears about the days ahead after that. Well, not any huge fears that overwhelmed us. The gratitude of God sparing our children transcended even the mighty fear of having triplets.

Three of everything

So, on we went! Becky continued with the shots; I worked as many hours as I could, and we slowly started thinking about what we would need to take care of three babies at once. Becky joined POTATO, the Parents of Twins and Triplets club. She attended the meetings, got a mentor who had her own triplets, and started working on logistics. Man, I miss that; she had a knack for planning and preparation that I sadly lack! I am wonderful in unexpected situations when quick thinking and flexibility are required, so we made a good team. Three of everything other than one changing table—three chairs, three cribs, three blankies, and so many diapers!

Becky enjoyed most of the physical changes except for a month of nausea. She was SO proud of her baby bump which eventually grew to a mound! Becky was tall, 5'10", and not a dainty lady. She had been back-up center for her high school basketball team, and we both enjoyed a good meal. But maintaining three babies in-utero took its toll in terms of her being tired and losing weight. It was never an issue, but she did love the way her face looked when she lost some extra pounds. She was so cute as her tummy grew, until it got to be difficult to move around and get in and out of the car. That was difficult. She would sometimes cry that she was fat and I would tell her she was not fat; she was a champion among women, preparing to birth triplets! Nothing for a wimpy woman to attempt, only for an Amazon such as her. While I would do it with a joke, she appreciated the support and knowing I was so proud of her, which I was.

Ah, the names. One name was spoken for, as I am Thomas Cornelius Monroe III. So one of the boys was going to be quart, I mean the fourth. I lobbied for Quart as a nickname to no avail. Thomas Cornelius Monroe IV was given. That left naming rights for two more. We thought of a lot of names for our daughter. I have the list of names Becky was trying out in her organized way. Melody, Laurel, and Lauren were the leading contenders.

Becky decided on Lauren, and we added Elizabeth for the Christian connotations and as a tribute to Becky's mother and Becky herself whose name was Rebecca Elizabeth Peter. Her last name gave me the idea for Peter Martin Monroe. That, and Peter was always my favorite apostle.

Martin came from my mother's maiden name. And it flowed. It was important to me how the names sounded together, and all three worked that way for me.

But then we needed to decide which boy was which. At first, I was thinking we would make the firstborn my namesake. But as I continued to consider that, I did not want Peter to feel any slight or difficulty from the firstborn son being named for my family. So, a week or so before their birth, we changed the order. Peter would be the first boy and Thomas the second. I am not sure what we were so concerned about as about 10 minutes separated their birth; so in the scheme of things, firstborn is really just a participation trophy.

We wondered how long she could carry them. Full term was not in our sights, but we hoped they'd make it to eight months. Her cervix began to thin a bit early so she got a cerclage to help with that. And we both went to the doc appointments, which were too much for one person to deal with. We had an ultrasound scheduled for October 24 to see how everyone was doing. I left work a little early to be there when I got a surprise call from her. "Trey, get here soon honey. We are going to be parents today."

Somehow, I managed to get the car parked without incident. I rushed up to her hospital room; she had been admitted and I saw the flurry of activity as the hospital folks prepared for the big game.

"What's going on?"

"It's Thomas. He has an infection and his water broke. We need to induce."

Becky was really quite afraid, and I did what I always did in those circumstances: I presented myself as the epitome of confidence. I think things were happening too fast for me to be concerned or stressed, but I did know what role would support Becky. Her mother was there, having transported Becky. So they wheeled her away and I got in my scrubs and joined her in the delivery room. There was barely room for me in there.

If my memory serves, there were 27 folks in the room, not counting triplets. In truth, there were a few extra people there to watch. The pace was quick once the party started. Thank you doctors, nurses, janitors, technicians, and observers.

Becky was comfortable during the process, her OB/GYN was a champ, and Lauren was born first. The entire delivery took about nine minutes between first-born Lauren and third-born Thomas. What an amazing technical achievement! I get tearful writing this because it was the most amazing event of my life. I had been present for the birth of Mary, but that was a typical pregnancy and delivery. This was not. Nowhere close. Lauren was so lovely, she breathed on her own but did not cry much. I touched her briefly, and she was whisked away to be cared for.

Next, about five minutes later, came Peter. He was the largest of the three, a couple ounces over three pounds. He too was calm and comfortable and was quickly escorted to be attended to. Almost as soon as Peter was gone, there came Thomas. And he cried the most pitiful cry I had ever heard, his lower jaw shaking from the effort. But he looked fine, and I had no worries about any of them.

I was escorted out, back to the room, and waited for my Becky to be brought back in. She was frustrated that I had seen them better than she had, but otherwise woozy and inebriated from the meds. She deserved a nice buzz after what she had been through. After a bit, we went to gaze at them through the glass of the nursery, and came back to the room to unwind.

Then the neonatal pediatrician and our own pediatrician for our older daughter, Mary, came into the room. They both had the most broken effect and sad faces I had ever seen. It was horrifying. They sat down and asked me to sit down. Thomas, they said, was very ill from his infection and would likely not survive the night.

More miracles

I sobbed and felt a depth of despair and sadness I have only felt once since. Becky was spared from this, as she was in a happy dream land from the meds. I am thankful that my wife was spared that ordeal. I, on the other hand, had to go home alone. I called all the prayer warriors I knew and informed them of the situation. I spread out face down on my bed, with my knees on the floor, and begged my Lord and Savior for my son's life. Again, I cannot even write this without tears. I slept some that night, but suffered more.

The next day I got back to the hospital, checked on Becky who was recovering well, and asked about Thomas, expecting the worst. But that is the thing about expectations; they are just guesses in the dark. Thomas had rallied in the night. I celebrated with Becky who really did not understand why we were celebrating as she had been protected from the worst of it. And in a few hours I got to help bathe them, 1, 2, 3. Again, Becky was jealous!

The triplets spent five weeks in the Neonatal Intensive Care Unit, and we spent an hour a day there. Those wonderful nurses and techs and doctors and cleaning tech and others made sure our precious, tiny souls were safe.

A community of support

The next few months and years call for many thank you's for various groups of heroes.

First up in the gratitude timeline, Nashville Fertility Center. At first they could not help us, but they took a chance in telling us of the new technology and hope that was made possible with embryo donation and our ability to "adopt" these precious embryos.

Of course, we owe a big thank you to the Neonatal Intensive Care Unit at St. Joseph Hospital in Nashville.

This next thank you involved so many people. After Becky was pregnant then gave birth to three babies, we had the ups and downs of the process and worrying about how in the world we could care for three infants at the same time. People have asked how two people raise triplets plus an older child; we did not. WE HAD HELP! Thank you, God, for the people who helped and supported us as we raised a quartet.

God sent angels of support and love to help us through. There was my dear Mother-in-law, Jean Peter. She provided immeasurable help with so many things during the pregnancy. There was our Pastor Tom Lovell, and the other folks at Bellevue Presbyterian Church. We would have truly collapsed under exhaustion and stress but for our church family.

When the triplets were infants, folks from church came over to care for them so Becky could take a shower. They brought food. They brought packages of diapers. They brought everything we needed.

Our friends Tom and Patty, and our dear friend Cathy Matthews who was fighting for her own cancer recovery but had energy to cheer us on at the same time! My family, mom and dad, and Fay and James

Kohoutek were there to lift us up as well.

Our friends and neighbors at Christ Presbyterian Church were also amazing to us. We camped in the third row of the sanctuary as the triplets grew up, wanting them to be close to the action. Becky and I taught Wednesday night classes at church and got to know the other kids and parents. Todd Teller and other staff and friends provided counsel and support through tough times. While they were not present for the baby part of the journey, they helped shape the character and spiritual lives of our children. Our gratitude is full for this congregation and how they love us!

And now thanks for the big sister role, Mary Bedford Monroe Hausfeld. Mary Bedford, circumstances gave you a not-so-easy road in your family life, and you were resilient. What a great blessing to us all. And lastly: our triplets all started here: In the hearts of this Christian couple who knew that their "extra" embryos were life and holy and deserved protection. Words fail to express the gratitude I feel toward Chris and Brooke Martin. May God bless you half as much as you blessed us.

Triplet toddler years

The next few months and years were busy, stressful, and very entertaining. We lived in an 1800-square-foot, two-story townhome with all of the bedrooms upstairs. During the day, our downstairs living room became the central location for the triplets, with a plastic gate providing containment. Our dining room table was converted to a changing table. Our galley-style kitchen produced an incredible amount of food over the years. As the triplets grew into toddlers, they loved running outside in the shared space between the townhomes. One tree in particular became the favorite climbing tree. We had several neighbors asking if we could get them to stop climbing the tree, and we would respond that we would love the help to get that done.

The whole time, despite the juggle and stress, Becky absolutely adored being a mother. When the triplets were born, one of the nurses in the delivery room was an amazing RN named Libby. Over time, Libby and her husband Chris became our dear friends, spending hours at our house pouring love into our crazy family.

So many similarities!

As the biological mom, I couldn't get enough information about the triplets' childhood and upbringing. The more I spoke with Trey and the kids, the more I realized how alike our families were. Like me, Becky stayed home with her babies until they started kindergarten. Becky was also the corporate breadwinner, so a lot of planning and sacrificing had to be made financially. I also learned more about the Monroe triplets as babies and toddlers, and there were moments I felt both entertained and guilty that they were very "active" as toddlers. I have apologized, with humor, for the shenanigans that the triplets must have caused. I cannot even imagine the feeling of managing the three spinning plates that were their busy toddlers.

One story of the triplets has been retold many times. Trey and Becky planned a much-needed evening out so hired a babysitter. The kids were still in diapers but were very mobile. At the time, the family dining table—located adjacent to the family room—doubled as a changing table. The table was glass so as one baby was getting changed, others would play underneath. Apparently when diaper-changing time was needed that night, Thomas displayed his coordination by taking his diaper off and painting the table with its contents. At the same time, the other two toddlers observed and followed suit. This led to mass chaos as well as a huge mess. When Trey and Becky returned home, they were both horrified and entertained. With their problem-solving minds, the only thing that seemed to work was to use duct tape instead of the flimsy diaper tape so that their creative triplets couldn't remove their diapers. The story is now referred to as "The Diaper Incident."

Trey and Becky, like us, took great care in making sure that each child had their own identity and opportunities to shine. Each child developed their own hobbies, and each had their own talents. Many of those talents and hobbies, we discovered, paralleled those of Christopher and Matthew's.

Out of the three, Peter seemed to be closest to his mom. None of the kids were jealous about this fact, and all agree that Peter has a gentle spirit. He is loyal, spiritual, and a deep thinker. Peter played sports for a while and dabbled in playing piano, but he most enjoyed video games. When Becky died, he seemed to look inward for answers. When learning about the Martin connection, Peter took longer to reflect on the big picture of the effect this might have on the relationship with his father and siblings.

Thomas—the baby who almost died in the hours after his birth—thrived in competitive sports. After playing football in middle school, he settled into wrestling in high school, winning many awards. He proved to be a go-getter, receiving his associates degree in History after high school while working, and becoming a personal trainer.

By the time she was in sixth grade, Lauren discovered her voice and showed incredible natural ability. Trey also has musical talent, but more in the way of an obsession with the history of musicians, so the very dominant musical ability in Lauren was always interesting. Trey and Becky wondered if it was a genetic trait or something she learned in her youth. From a very young age, she could memorize the exact pitch of a song and be able to repeat it hours and even days later. She would correct anyone on the pitch and rhythm of a song. By the time she was in high school, she was singing solos in church and in choir at school, and she loved playing the guitar.

Learning about their biological origin

Lauren recalls they had knowledge that Becky had to go through some kind of fertility treatments to give birth to them and said she always felt compassion and gratitude that her mom went to great lengths to have them. She recalls that she never felt adopted or that she didn't belong. But at some point, the reality that they weren't biologically related became more real. At the age of 13 or 14, Peter asked the question about the biological relationship between the triplets and his parents. Trey and Becky explained the science to them, like we did to our boys. But they also stressed that all three children were created by God and appointed to be in the Monroe family. They always felt loved and included, and no different than a biological child would.

According to Lauren, Trey and Becky explained that they weren't their biological parents in a way that made it seem like they were miracles. They were reminded about this throughout their lives so that when they met their biological family, there would be a positive association with it.

A huge piece of our story is the fact that Trey was reunited with his biological family in 2016. He knew he was adopted from a young age, so he decided to do an Ancestry.com search. He then found his first cousin, Brooke Thorington, who lived in Louisiana. The fact that he found another "Brooke" is another of the ironic coincidences. With Brooke Thorington's help, Trey was able to find his biological mother and siblings—the Ball family. This extended family has provided the Monroes very meaningful relationships over the years, as the family that raised him had already passed away.

As our story unfolded, members of the Ball family, including Brooke Thorington, reached out to me on social media to express their amazement. Now I consider the Ball family an extended part of our family, and I realize that the definition of "family" is that of acceptance, love, and recognition of the beauty that God created within our complicated story.

The diagnosis

In 2018, during a routine doctor's visit, Becky discovered that she had colorectal cancer. The triplets were 16 and already experiencing grief from watching their Aunt Katie die from a brain tumor.

Becky and Trey told their children around the dinner table, with the knowledge that "this is not Katie's cancer." The plan of treatment was simple but would disrupt Becky's organized schedule for the family: chemo followed by radiation. According to the doctors, the cancer had been caught early and had a high probability of being treated effectively. All this while having 16-year-old triplets at home, trying to navigate high school.

Lauren remembers coming home from school and talking to Becky about her school day, and watching her nod off to sleep due to exhaustion from the cancer treatment.

After her first round of treatments that year, Becky's cancer went into remission. But less than a year later, it came back and had spread to other parts of her body. Her deterioration from there was rapid, and treatments were unsuccessful.

Becky lost her battle with cancer on January 24, 2020. Her precious triplets were 17 years old and juniors in high school.

DNA search

On the triplets 18th birthday, October 24, 2020, nine months after his mother's death, Thomas asked Trey if he could get a DNA test to find out about his biological lineage. I imagine that if Trey had a negative experience in finding his biological family, Thomas' request for a DNA kit would not have been met with such positivity, and the story would have had a much different outcome.

At the time there were two main DNA search companies—Ancestry.com and 23andMe. Trey decided to buy what he thought was the least likely choice of DNA kits: 23andMe. Ancestry.com was the more popular DNA kit at the time. He said he was fine with them finding their biological roots, but a small part of him didn't want a complicated outcome to navigate. In reality, either of the DNA tests would have found multiple members of the Martin extended family and eventually led to the origin of the adopted embryos. By mid-November, Thomas received the results back and started reaching out to one of the connections, named Tod McCoy, and the communication started.

Our Love Multiplied

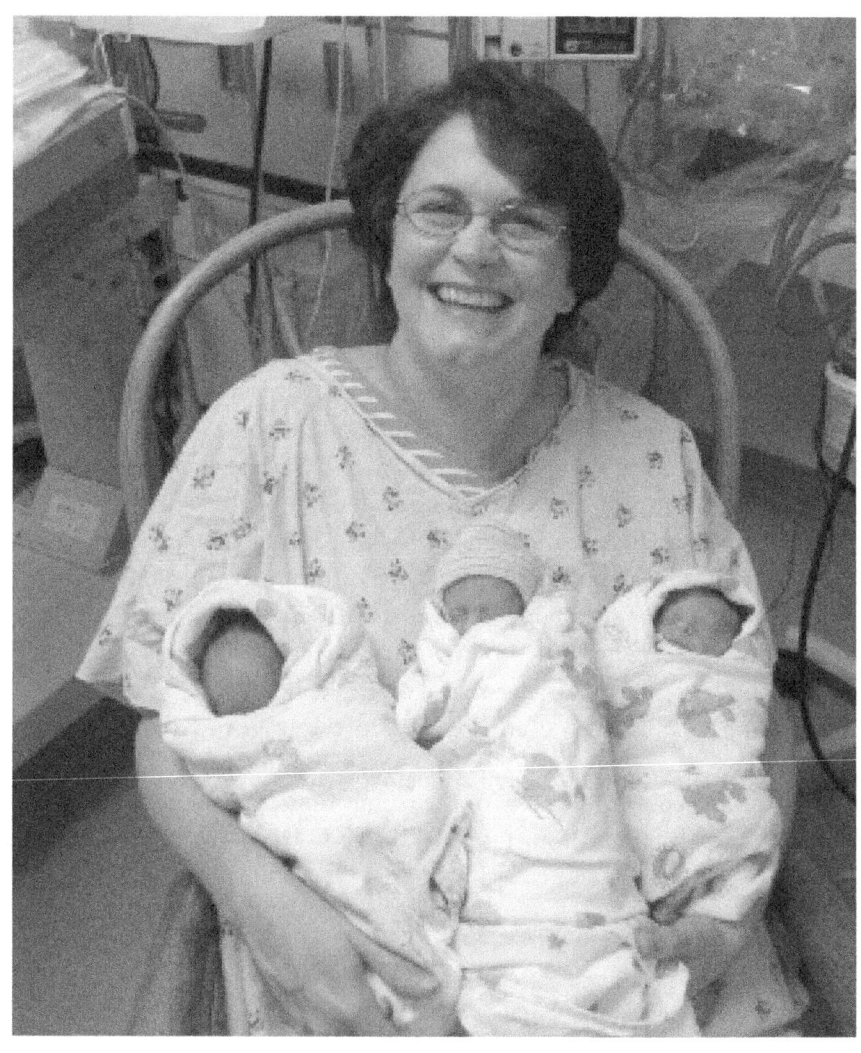

Becky Monroe with newborn triplets.

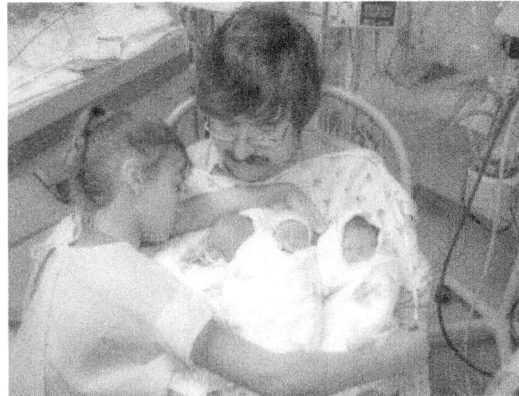

Trey and newborn triplets with sister Mary.

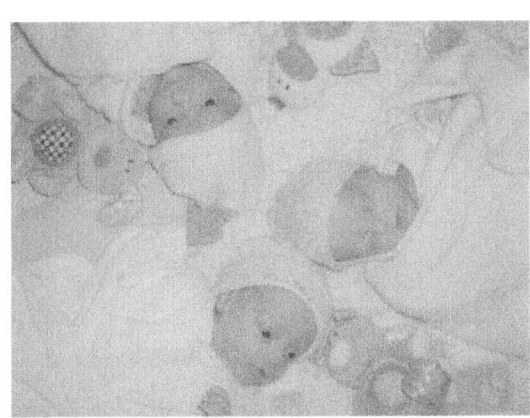

The Monroe triplets.

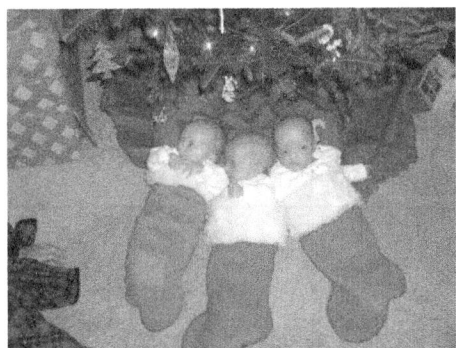

The Monroe's Christmas stockings, December 2022.

Thomas (L), Peter (M), and Lauren (R).

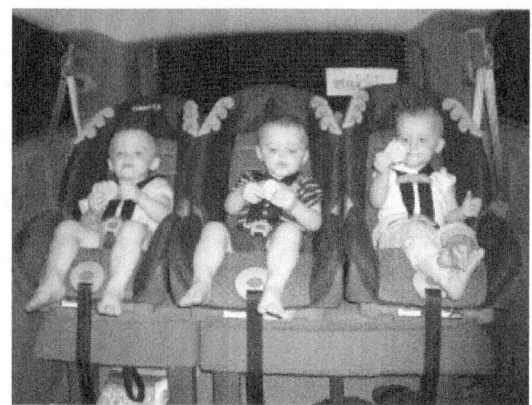

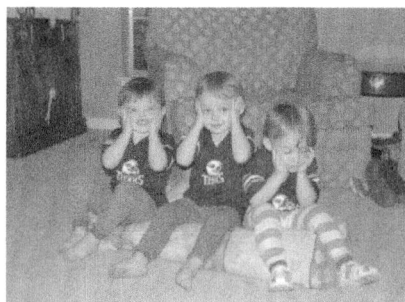

The Monroe triplets being silly. Peter (L), Thomas (M), and Lauren (R).

The Monroe triplets roughhousing.

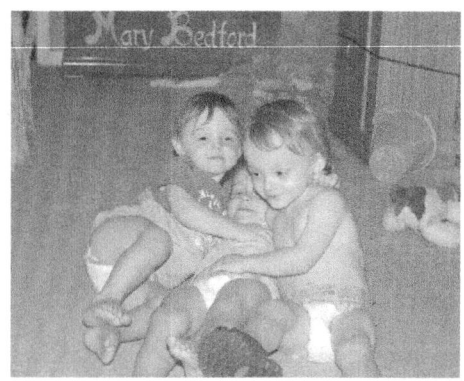

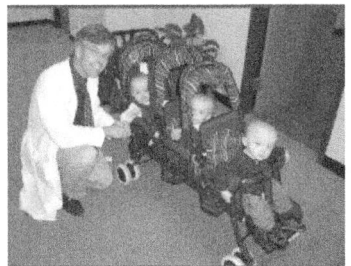

Triple stroller with Dr. Geoffrey H. Smallwood, the OB/GYN who delivered the triplets.

Lauren (L), Thomas (M), and Peter (R).

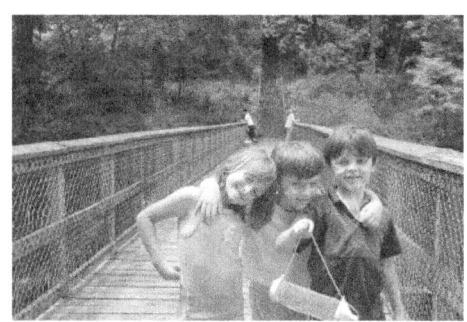

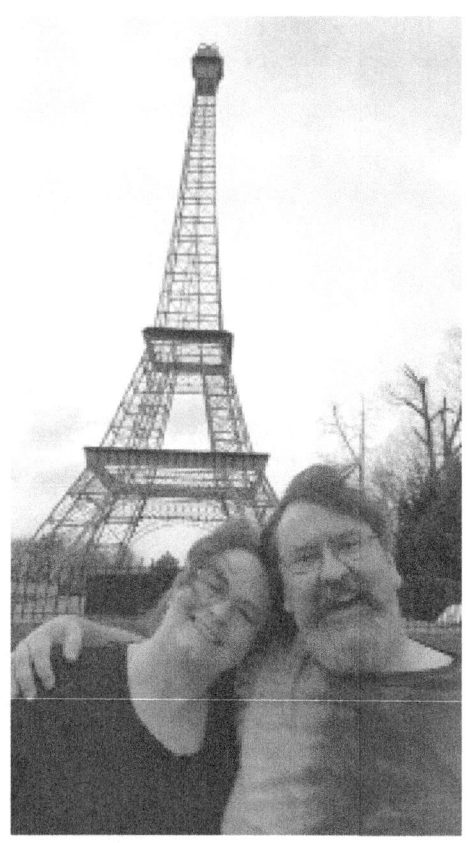

Becky and Trey Monroe at Eiffel Tower Park in Paris, TN (2010).

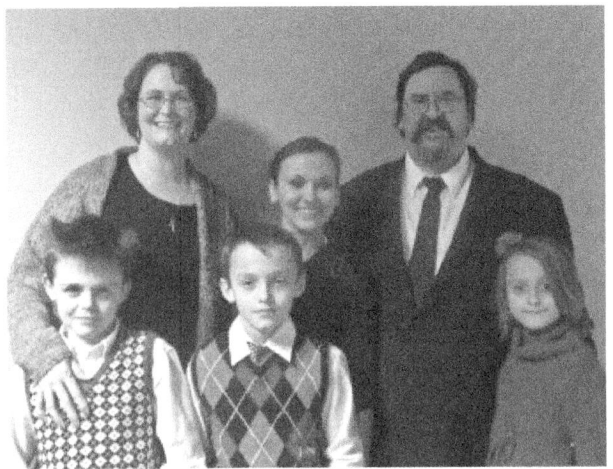

The Monroe family. Back row: Becky and Trey Monroe with sister Mary. Front row: Peter (L), Thomas (M), and Lauren (R) (2010).

Part 4—The Meeting

Within the first couple of months of the January 2021 emails, the topic of a face-to-face meeting entered every conversation between Trey and us. Inside my head, I was SO incredibly excited about that possibility. But I didn't want to be overbearing.

Trey soon mentioned that he would encourage his kids to meet their "Texas family." This concept had a huge impact on me. My husband and I and my two boys had been a very nuclear family for many years. Both of our sets of parents had passed away, so it had been just the four of us since the boys were in middle school. We had moved around the country together and had experienced life without consistent contact with cousins, aunts and uncles. But when we found out about Trey's story of adoption and finding his biological family, Chris and I felt that the comfort level of our developing relationships made it possible for us to consider meeting them.

Trey's openness about his and Becky's journey: marrying later in life, experiencing the pain of infertility, then having the opportunity for Becky to realize her dream of pregnancy and motherhood, always brings tears to my eyes. I felt so incredibly blessed that such an amazing, God-fearing couple adopted our embryos and raised them in an environment similar to ours. For Trey to be supportive of his children meeting us was more than I could have ever asked for. For that and the friendship we have developed with Trey, we will always be grateful.

The first meeting

Our son Christopher had met Nora, the love of his life, at the end of high school. After living in separate cities and trying to date during Covid, they decided they wanted to get married. After a beautiful Thanksgiving Day proposal in 2020, they were married in March 2021 during the height of the Covid separation. Due to travel restrictions, there were only seven family members in attendance at their wedding—but it was a joyous day! They decided that when Covid subsided, they would have a wedding celebration the following summer and would invite relatives from out of town and possibly from out of state. One day when planning the summer 2021 event, they excitedly asked if they could invite the Monroes.

I was surprised and touched that they wanted to open the invitation to the triplets. I didn't want to overshadow their celebration, but I was thrilled at the thought of having all of the biological kids together. I was also imagining how overwhelmed the Monroe kids might be at the size and volume of the Martin family!

Almost immediately, Thomas and Lauren were on board with making the trip to Texas for the celebration. We knew that Peter wasn't quite ready to meet, and that was fine. Thomas said that he would "check to make sure we were OK people," then hopefully Peter would be willing to at least meet us in the future.

The day that Thomas and Lauren flew to Houston, Matthew was there with us to greet them at the airport. Although I was nervous about meeting them, I also felt that this was both the closing of a circle and an opening of a beautiful new chapter of our story. When the two came down the escalator to the baggage claim area to meet us, my first reaction was surprise; I noticed that Thomas had the same gait as both Matthew and my brother. In fact, meeting Thomas was almost uncomfortable because he looked SO much like my brother…with some Matthew and Christopher thrown in there.

Although Lauren has my personality, and we share the same expressions, I immediately realized how much she looks like Christopher—the same jawline and the same smile. She also looked a lot like me when I was her age.

Chris was worried about coming on too strong; he has a big personality and often makes unfiltered comments. Even though we weren't their parents, our parental instincts kicked in. We wanted to learn about them so we could help encourage them. We wanted them to be successful in their lives. But they have a father—a very good one—and we were very aware to respect Trey. As far as my urge to "mother" them, that was a tough balance. Even though their mom wasn't there, I did not want to be perceived as wanting to take her place. I wasn't sure what that would look like, but I was just overjoyed to meet them in person!

The plan was for the Monroe kids to ride with us to Waco since our car couldn't hold three adults in the back seat, then Matthew would drive separately. The trip was close to three hours long.

On the ride from Houston to Waco, there was constant chatter. I don't even remember what we talked about, but I know there was no silence. They were getting ready to meet A LOT of family, but they both seemed positive about their decisions to be there for the occasion. I purposefully didn't want to start referring to them in conversations as "the one that looks like Matthew" or "the one that also sings." They are all unique individuals who have already had 18 years of life to discover their talents, their dreams, and their individualities. But it was hard to not make comparisons; even they kept bringing up the similarities between them and their newfound brothers.

When we arrived at the hotel in Waco on Friday evening, there were lots of family members already there. Thomas and Lauren met not only Christopher but also cousins, aunts, and uncles. The adults gathered together and were catching up while all the kids were also together talking. My master plan was for all of us to go to dinner and break the ice, making it easier for the kids to get to know each other.

Many people ask if Chris and I had an immediate connection to the Monroe triplets. I think we did, but even more surprising was the immediate connection they all had with my sons, their biological brothers. Even as I was talking with the adults, my eyes were constantly shifting over to watch how the kids were interacting. I could tell that relationships were blooming.

Within 30 minutes of the initial meeting in Waco, the four kids came over and told us they were heading down the street to get some tacos and would catch up with us later.

Just like that! There they went. So much for my master plan. I was shocked, but relieved.

Later that evening, Lauren and I spent time together and had lots of girl talk that I never thought I would have with a daughter. In my family, many of the women were full-figured. My maternal grandmother, Mabel Bonham, started the saying that women in the family had the "Bonham Butt," and we giggled about how she inherited that feature. She told me that she had always wondered where it came from. On Saturday morning, we went shopping for shorts because due to her curves, she was having trouble finding the right fit to look appropriate. I reminded her that finding shorts is challenging because clothing isn't made for women like us. It was fun discussing that similarity and helping her find clothes that fit her. She realized how different this experience was for me, and at one point asked, "So what's it like shopping with your daughter?"

Once again, I was surprised and speechless. My mind still didn't know what to do with the feelings that came with the new experience. I gave her a hug and said, "It's *very* different from shopping with my boys!"

She was such a beautiful young woman, yet I could tell she still needed guidance. She told me that since her mom passed away, she had mostly relied on her teenage friends for advice about things like buying clothes and how to survive as a young woman in the world. I had been given a very special gift to be in her life: the opportunity to soften my heart and influence a young woman who was my biological daughter. I wanted to do things right. I asked God then, and I continue to ask Him, how to give her the best advice and help carefully guide her in ways specific to her needs.

Lauren's personality was more confrontational than mine, and I was amused how she was able to hold her place in conversations with Chris when he would be sarcastic or direct. She told me that was because she was raised with two brothers and had to learn to stand up for herself. She showed she had a quick wit and was able to answer Chris' pointed comments.

One of Christopher's good friends from high school, Alex, alo came to the wedding celebration. They had spent much of their junior and senior years singing together both in choir and performing in restaurants around Houston. Christopher set up a keyboard at the reception the night before the celebration so that he and Alex could relive some memories. During the evening, Lauren was invited to sing with Christopher, and although she was nervous with all of the new family attending, there was magic in the air when her voice blended with Christopher's. My momma's heart was so full and still in some disbelief that this was happening. The room was full, and everyone was enjoying and accepting the new cousins.

The next day, Christopher and Nora's wedding celebration was at their church in downtown Waco. Many relatives had flown in for the celebration, including cousin Tod who had originally contacted us. Chris' brothers and sisters from Tennessee and North Carolina were there along with their spouses, including the B. Martin (Bret) that Thomas had found on 23andMe. I wanted to control everything and make sure everyone was comfortable and welcome, but it all happened so naturally.

The extended Martin family was so welcoming and loving, and I saw Lauren and Thomas having conversations with their newfound cousin Bryce, Bret's son. They all noticed they had the same high forehead and took a comparison picture by lifting their bangs up. We took a photo of all of the family who attended the wedding, with Lauren and Thomas joining. The Monroe kids blended into the family that weekend…their "Texas family" as Trey had said. It was a surreal experience, and it was perfect. I didn't have to "do" anything to create love and acceptance. It was family.

There were many hugs and surprised looks when family members saw all of the similarities with the Monroe kids and the Martin boys. At one point I took a picture of Matthew and Thomas. I said "smile boys," and they made the exact same faces. That kind of thing happened a lot in Waco that weekend. Thomas and Matthew were so similar in so many ways. They walked ahead of me on the sidewalk and their gait was absolutely identical. I took a video of them walking side-by-side, and it was so mind-blowing that I exclaimed, "Stop it! Y'all are hysterical!"

After the wedding celebration, we drove back to our house in Humble, Texas, and spent time looking at Martin family pictures. Chris told the Monroe kids about his family who had lived in

Nashville two generations ago and how they owned a saloon downtown. We had found some historical pictures of the family and shared them with Lauren and Thomas. They were genuinely interested in the details of their genealogy, which proved that the relationship between us and the Monroe kids would continue.

That night, Lauren and Thomas slept upstairs in Christopher and Matthew's old bedrooms. I hesitated before doing that, but it was more a feeling of, "am I doing the right thing"? It was another foreign thought for my brain to process: my recently-found biological children are now sleeping in the beds that my adult twin boys slept in during high school.

After that initial meeting, I kept in touch with both Lauren and Thomas, but of course wanted to meet Peter and Trey. When we lived in Tennessee, we were Tennessee Titans football fans and had attended almost every home game until I was too pregnant to make the trip to Nashville. So, we got tickets to go to a Titans game for us and the Monroe's in August 2021.

Trey had made plans to meet us at the Loveless Café in Belleview, Tennessee, the day we arrived. I was very nervous to meet him. There were no words to adequately say what I wanted to express, so I decided that small talk was going to have to suffice for our first meeting. We drove up and parked, and I got out of the car to see a very friendly smile from a big burly man that had lovingly raised my biological children. There was an immediate understanding between us.

We talked over breakfast about the struggles we all went through with infertility, and I asked many questions about what the triplets were like as babies, toddlers, and teenagers. From the first day we met, Trey had a sense of humor that brought a lightness to our situation which helped tremendously. He told us stories that morning about the duct taping diapers incident, stories about the insanity of having triplet babies, and stories about what a blessing they have been to him. Many times I was laughing, shaking my head and apologizing humorously for the genes that were passed down, saying "so sorry they were so wild!" He also reminded us how Becky loved them so dearly. My cup of gratitude was filled up and running over!

Later that day, we had plans for Lauren and her boyfriend, and Peter and his girlfriend, to meet us at the Titans Stadium. I was nervous about meeting Peter, concerned that he might see me as a threat to the close relationship he had with his mother. My childhood friend Tracey and her husband were tailgating with friends, so we showed up a little early to hang out with them. While they were talking, I was pacing and looking at the entry road, and distracted with the upcoming reunion.

The traffic getting into the stadium was hard to navigate, and with only 10 minutes before kickoff, the Monroe crew still had not arrived. Lauren was sending me texts on their ETA, and Chris was worried we would miss the beginning of the game. When they finally arrived, everyone was walking at a fast pace to get through the gate, so the initial meeting was a quick hug and hello. Looking back, I'm glad that the meeting was in public and we had to keep moving. As we got to our seats in the nosebleed section, Peter sat next to Chris, and Lauren sat next to me. I was very pleased to see Chris and Peter engaged in some small talk, and I felt the mood relax as the game started. Chris and Peter talked about the pizza business and chatted about the football game as it was starting.

Peter was, and still is, a soft-spoken young man. When I met him, I couldn't help but stare and notice all of the similarities between him and my boys. The same look of Matthew, the grin from Chris' side of the family. And many other features, including a thick head of wavy brown hair that he was growing out past his shoulders. I had a million questions to ask and so did he, so we had a great conversation that night. Although he was soft-spoken, we talked about his job and the ironic fact that Chris was also in the pizza industry. He really enjoyed the food service business and hoped to continue there. We talked about Christopher and Matthew, and we shared pictures of them at different ages. We thanked him for coming to meet us and let him know that we hope to continue getting to know each other. He told us that he figured he would meet us since Thomas and Lauren said we were good people. That made me feel so good! Even though the Titans lost, we took pictures with lots of smiles.

The next day, Lauren and Daniel decided to join us at our Nashville hotel rooftop pool. As we were chatting, the conversation turned to how to achieve life goals. Chris and I were able to give some advice about jobs, housing, and how to be independent adults. Lauren was still living at home and struggling to find a solid job, and her boyfriend was looking for direction. I realized again that God had also brought all of us together to help with these big decisions.

During our conversations with Trey and the kids, we recognized several other things that the families had in common, and one big similarity was eating good food—and lots of it! Whether it was sushi, barbeque, crawfish, or anything adventurous, both the Martins and Monroes would devour it.

The day after the Titan's game, we all met at the Monroe's favorite sushi restaurant. Most people are quite picky when it comes to eating sushi, but not this group. We ordered the family sushi boat, several bowls of edamame, and then Peter got several sides of sashimi. The amount of sushi we ate that night was astonishing.

During that same visit, Lauren and I decided to video record a conversation about our relationship in order to share it with others. By this time, we were both very open about how unique and special our chemistry was. Since Becky had been sick from the time Lauren was close to 16, there was "mom advice" that she sadly missed. Finding out that she had a biological mother felt like a healing that God had sent her. Even though losing her mom didn't make sense, finding me was a way for her to get closure.

At first, I felt like I could talk to Peter and Thomas better than Lauren since I had raised boys. But there I was, with my biological daughter who was asking me for advice about boys and being a woman. It was about this time that our relationship evolved from that of a friendship or one between an aunt and her niece. I felt like I'd become a mother figure. That summer, I was talking to Lauren on FaceTime while she was walking with some friends. They were being loud in the background and she said "y'all be quiet, I'm talking to my mom." It stunned me. I literally couldn't talk.

I continue to be surprised about how all three of the kids accepted us. Individually, they have been able to open up to me about personal things. It is more than I could have ever hoped for. I have to credit that to Trey, who has encouraged open communication, has expanded the definition of "family," and has reminded us to follow our heart instead of any arbitrary rules. Except there are no rules for this. Hopefully we can help others going through the same circumstance know what to do. We have followed our gut instincts, sometimes being fearless, and moving ahead with those instincts. There have been many times when Lauren asked my advice, and I wanted to give her some honest truth. I thought about it, prayed about it, and did what I thought was right. It has been a big responsibility, and I have taken it very seriously.

The question of "nature versus nurture" always comes up in conversation when we talk about our story. The fact is, the Monroe family and the Martin family were very similar in many ways, including the way each family disciplined and expected appropriate behaviors from their children. Our belief system as strong Christians was complementary, but neither group was stuffy or judgmental about it. Trey has always enjoyed a good cigar and some fine bourbon, and we enjoy happy hour frequently. Becky was not the typical quiet, stay-at-home mom, and I have been a corporate worker for many years.

Both couples' faith in God has been tested and tried, and we have all proved that God is faithful and has a sense of humor. That reflection and honesty with all of the children resulted in them having similar attitudes toward life and toward God. Thomas was kind, driven and although not religious, he has respect for those around him. Peter's experience with faith led to deep truths that were challenged by his mother's death. But during the next couple of years, he and I had some discussions about God's plan for his life. Lauren's fiery personality also included a deep faith in God with insight into the spiritual significance of our story.

I can see glimpses of Thomas in Matthew, similarities between Lauren and Christopher, and the softness of Peter reflected in all of the kids.

Family reunion

In the fall of 2021, I was able to go to Nashville on a work trip and visit again with Lauren. We'd started talking and texting on a regular basis—maybe once a week—and discussing things like boyfriends, daily struggles, and commiserating on not being able to find any clothes meant for women with a few extra curves. We also discovered that we both had a love for big sunglasses, and I loved putting together "comparison pics" for the Love Multiplied Facebook page.

In April of 2022, we found out that the Martin family in Tennessee was planning a family reunion in July, and it happened to fall on the same weekend as Chris' 40th high school reunion. We thought it would be a great time for the Monroe kids to meet the rest of the Martin family, and in my romantic "hope of all hopes" heart, I wanted all five of the kids to be there.

It was at this point that the complexities of planning an event with this newfound five-offspring family became painfully obvious. We were unsure if Christopher and Nora would be able to come since they lived in Waco. In addition, Matthew had enlisted in the US Navy in January 2022 and was now living in Charleston, SC, going to school to be a Naval Nuclear Mechanic. With that much advanced planning, Christopher and Nora were "in" and excited about it. I pitched the idea carefully to Trey, since Lauren and Peter were still living at home. His answer, again, shook me. He said "I will make sure that all three of the kids are there to meet their family!"

Then...the icing on the cake: Matthew could ask for a long weekend off, drive to meet Chris' brother Bret in Charlotte, NC, and ride with him to the reunion.

The plan was in place: All three Monroe kids and Trey, my daughter-in-law, Chris and I, our two boys, and dozens of the Martin family!

The reunion was at my husband's brother Buck's house in Sparta, Tennessee. Chris and I arrived with Christopher and Nora, and there were cousins from Nashville that I hadn't seen in many years. Matthew showed up with Bret, his wife Gaynell, and their son Bryce. Matthew was in his green Naval uniform and looked so handsome. There were several cousins who had not heard about the "extra kids," until we arrived, and many others were anticipating the Monroe's arrival. When they drove up, I realized again that I was not in control and could not be privy to all of the conversations that were about to happen. Peter had not met either Christopher or Matthew, and Trey was also in the mix to explain how he raised biological Martin kids. I also wanted to spend time with Matthew and learn about nuclear power school, but I also wanted to be there to support Thomas, Peter, and Lauren.

Ok God, you are in control. Take the wheel!

But just like the Waco visit, the flow of conversations were smooth and natural. Lauren commented that she felt the "brother vibe" from all of the boys and definitely felt outnumbered more than ever before. My boys and the triplets were sitting in rocking chairs on the back porch of Buck's house, talking and cutting up. Buck had gone through family photos and sorted them by each branch of the Martin family. One table was full of pictures of Chris when he was a baby, his oldest sister Becky who carried him around when he was an infant, and of Chris' parents and grandparents. All five kids were fascinated with the family history, and the Monroe triplets were soaking in all of the information. Buck had set up tables in his covered garage for the family to enjoy a barbeque meal, complete with homemade potato salad and plenty of desserts. During the meal we watched a slideshow of family pictures, many of which Chris and I had never seen. The Monroe kids were part of the family now.

Going viral

I decided to talk to everyone at the family reunion about going public with our story. We had a lot of attention on our Facebook page and agreed that we loved watching the joy that our story brought to anyone who heard it. I wanted to find a Houston TV reporter who could tell our story in the right way—one who wasn't afraid or restricted to include our shared beliefs in the sanctity of life and the sovereignty of God. I also committed to the Monroes that every time the story was told, I would honor Becky.

Everyone was immediately on board.

So, in July, 2022 I started searching for the right person to break our story on a local news channel. I came across Melissa Wilson from Houston's Fox 26 when I saw that she had a weekly online story called "Lunch for the Soul" which devoted time to telling heart-felt, faith-rich stories. I reached out to her online and gave a synopsis of our story. Within a few days she answered, wanting more information. Melissa was and still is a strong Christian woman who lived not too far from us and has the sweetest demeanor. We started making plans to film but due to Covid restrictions, we did some filming at her house and pieced together some video from the kids online. She did a beautiful job with the interview and putting the story together in such a meaningful way. I was excited in anticipation of sharing our joy. The story aired in Houston on October 19, 2022, one day after my boys' 22nd birthday, and a week before the triplets turned 20.

That same day the story aired, it was decided the Houston Astros World Series were going to be playing at Minute Maid Park in Houston, so our story was actually bumped around in the news cycle and was considered second fiddle to the Minute Maid story. Being obsessed with the news overall, I followed the story once it was posted on the Fox26 website and tracked the number of likes or watches it had. Our story remained higher in the ratings than the Astros that week.

The next day, the morning of the 20th, my phone rang at 6 AM and startled me. It was Melissa with Fox26.

"I'm sorry to wake you up so early," she said quickly, "But your story has gone viral and I need your permission to release it to all of the major news channels. *Right now!*"

I scrambled out of bed, woke Chris up and told him the news. Melissa sent me a text that spelled out the need for me to give permission to release the story. I replied by text, "Permission given", then sat down on the edge of the bed. I looked at Chris and said,

"Well, here we go!"

Was I surprised that there was interest in our story? Not really. I was actually joyful. I knew our story would bring happiness to others. I received an email that day from News Nation and did an interview with them that week. Then I was contacted by CBS news online, and from there multiple online sources picked up the story and re-published it. The next few months were filled with emails from news outlets all over the world. We even found an article in Vietnamese!

I got the family's permission to be the main contact for the story, and if I felt like others needed to be looped in I would do that. I learned so much about the roller coaster of news cycles and the fact that "going viral" is like an online bomb going off. It's amazing how any news outlet or individual can pick up a story and sensationalize it to get clicks. Every once in a while, I will search my name and the words "embryo donation" on Google, and each time I am still amazed at seeing our story all over the world.

A few weeks after the story broke, I got an email from *Today. com*, the online version of NBC's *Today show*. We set up a phone interview and were able to get many of the kids involved for a printed story that was published online. A day or two after that story ran online in early November, I was connected with the producers of the *Today Show* who wanted to come film a segment on our story. They wanted some involvement from other family members and were willing to send a reporter and camera crew to Texas.

With Christopher living in Waco, we decided to find a place there to film so he could be involved, too. He had some friends there who had a beautiful house and spacious living room we could use for the interview. I was so nervous but also excited to share our story. The reporter was young and didn't know much about the IVF process, so I was able to explain our story to him and how the reunion happened. The home had a piano, and the camera man filmed Christopher playing the piano and then said he would add the video of him singing with Lauren. At one point during the interview, we were able to have Lauren and Trey join us on Facetime from Nashville so viewers could see us interact.

That Today Show interview was done on Saturday, November 19, the weekend before Thanksgiving. We thought it would be mixed in with the morning news sometime earlier in the week, but then we got word that our story was going to be featured on Thanksgiving morning, right before the Macy's Thanksgiving Day parade! It just was perfect timing. Our story of thankfulness and joy ! Once again, I was reminded that God's timing is perfect.

After the story aired, I received several phone calls and emails from surprised friends across the country. One work colleague that I didn't know well yet called me and asked how I was doing, then said, *"Did I just see you on the Today Show?"* The news was out!

Shortly after that, I got contacted by a reporter in the UK and learned all about how the media works there. It is very competitive, and they have "Mags," which are tabloids a little bit like *The National Inquirer* in the USA, but they are true stories that are magnified with drama. I did several interviews with them, including *The Daily Mail, The Daily Star, Closer,* and *That's Life*. Surprisingly, they all called me back and read the story to me in their sweet British accents for approval. In the United States, I was never asked for approval for any published articles.

Some of the "Mags" used flowery language, were overly emotional, and the scenes they created were fictional. But the facts were straight and the message was clear. Many of them did include our faith and our belief that life begins at conception. One of the articles had a headline of *"I met my triplets - 20 years after giving them away"*, but the one that tickled me the most had a headline of, *"I didn't know I had triplets!"* Their language was also different, saying that I "fell pregnant" and referring to me as "the mum". Several of them also sent me hard copies of the magazine which are now displayed in my office.

Although we have purposefully not taken a political stand, I had many people on social media claim that I had an agenda. There were a few negative comments on our Facebook page, but I had no problem responding with my belief system, which is not political at all. It is based on my life experience.

Shortly after the string of interviews and articles, I started to document our experiences and write this book. With the thought of a potential movie in the future, I felt the need to tell the story of both families in the most accurate way possible. It has taken more than two years to extract facts, and even more time to find words to attempt to express my thoughts and feelings as our story unfolded.

    Here is where some unanswered questions surface. The glaring question is: had anyone else adopted any of our other 5 embryos, and will we ever know? I remembered that we got some type of correspondence from the Nashville Fertility Center after we donated, asking us for more information. Upon getting the medical record, there was a letter dated August of 2001, requesting us to complete more information on our donor profile because someone was looking at the embryos. That was at least four months BEFORE the Monroe's were even presented with the option to adopt embryos. We don't know if some were adopted then or not. We may never know.

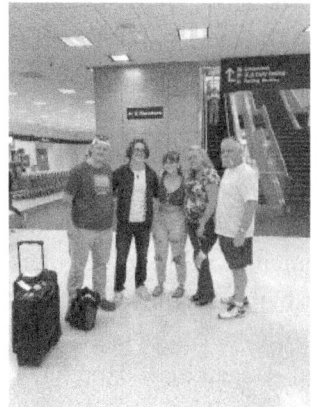

First meeting at the airport in Houston. (L-R) Matthew, Thomas, Lauren, Brooke, and Chris.

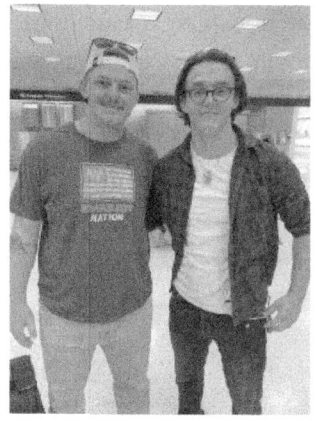

First meeting. Matthew (L) and Thomas (R).

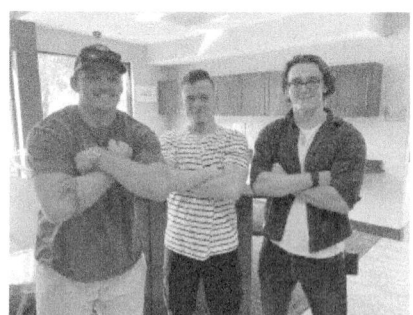

First meeting in Waco. (L-R) Matthew, Christopher, and Thomas.

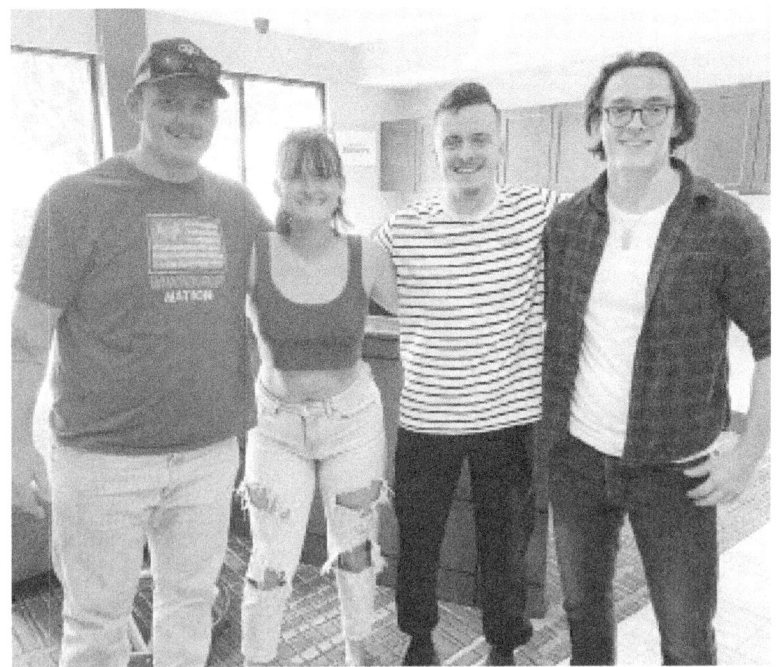

The first meeting in Waco. (L-R) Matthew, Lauren, Christopher, and Thomas.

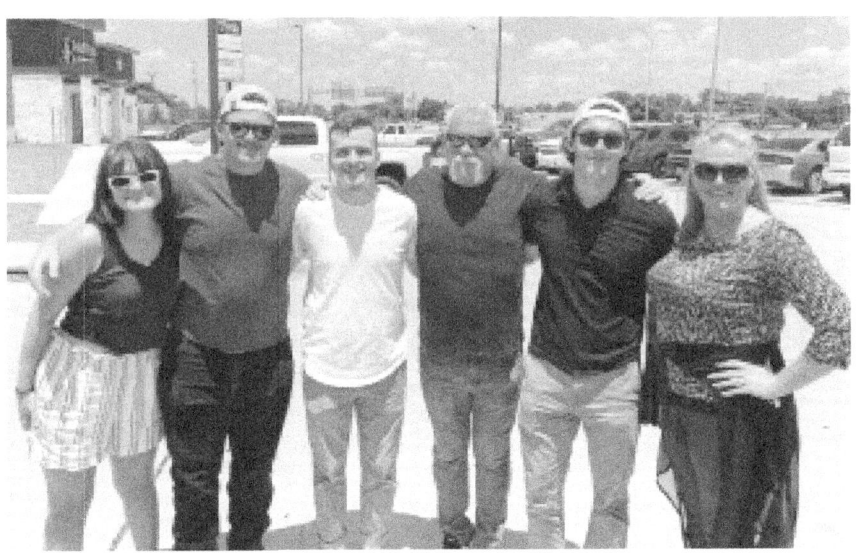

Together in Waco during the first meeting. (L-R) Lauren, Matthew, Christopher, Chris, Thomas, and Brooke.

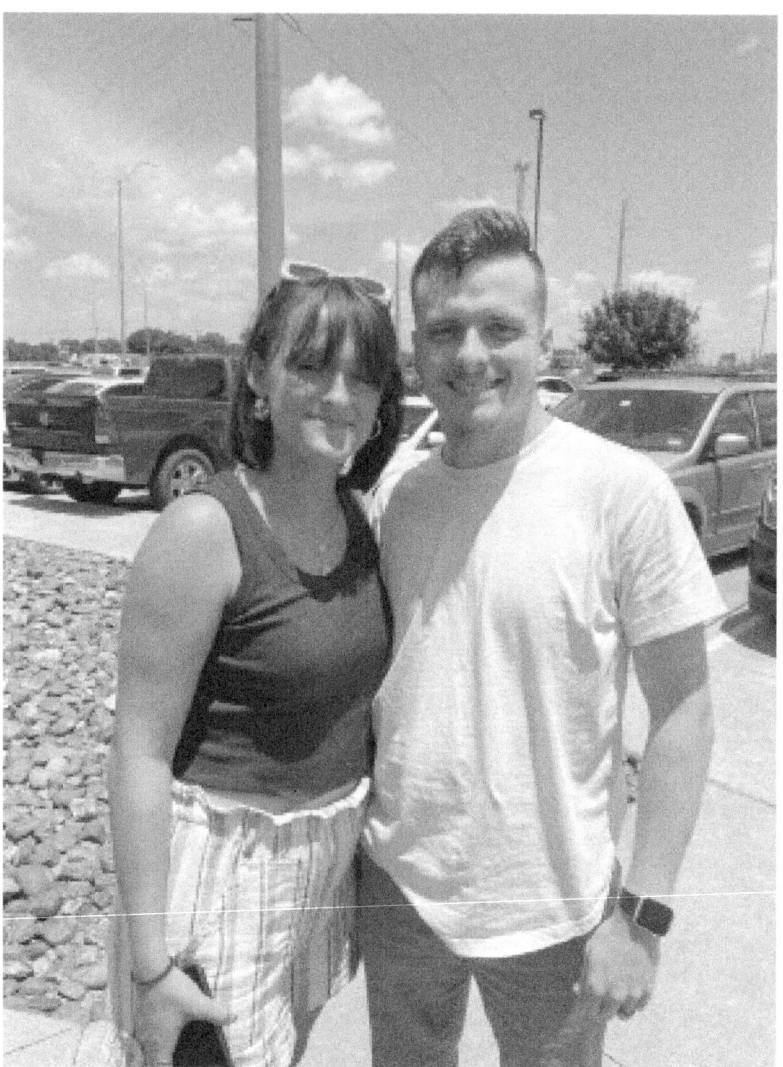
Sister and brother Lauren and Christopher at their first meeting.

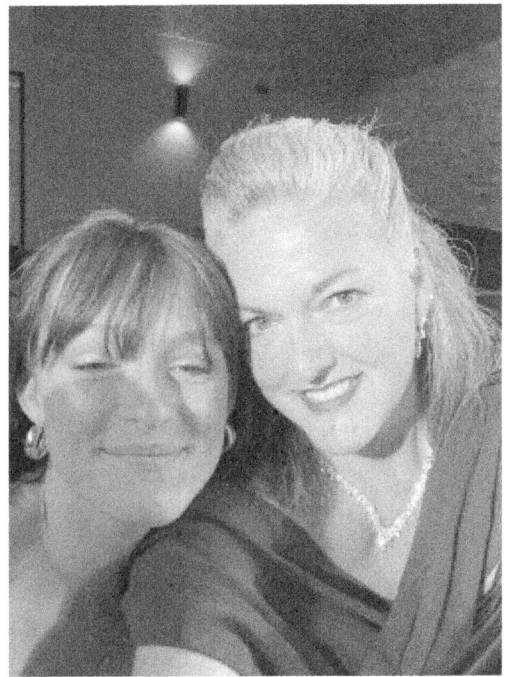
Lauren and Brooke at the wedding celebration.

Our Love Multiplied

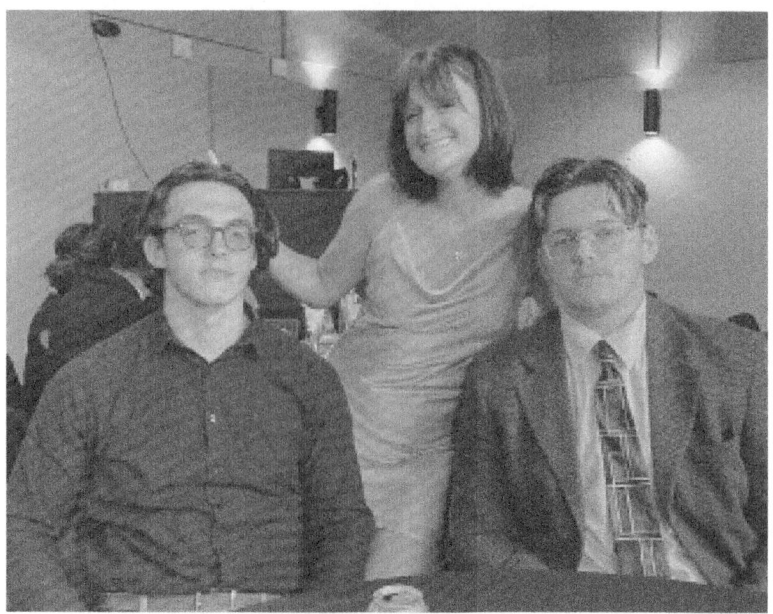

Thomas, Lauren, and Matthew at the wedding celebration when told to "smile", and the boys had the same expression.

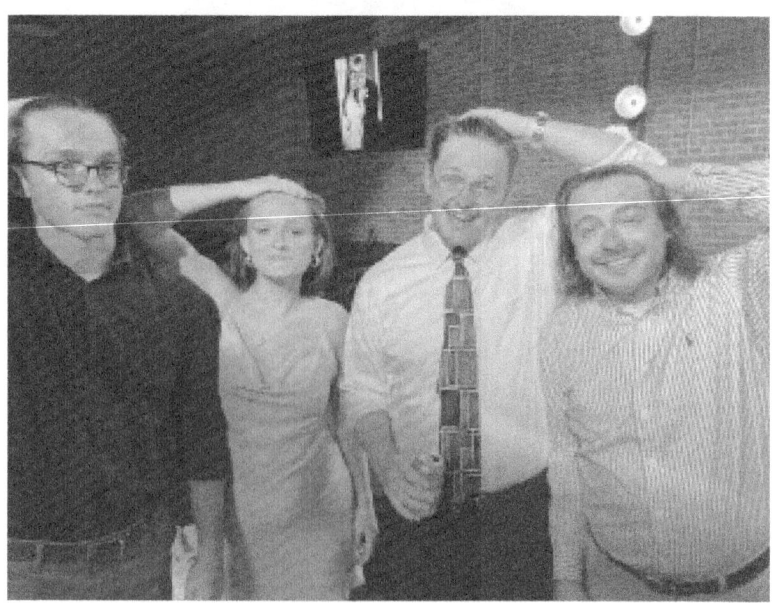

Comparing foreheads at the wedding celebration! (L-R), Thomas, Lauren, Matthew, and cousin Bryce.

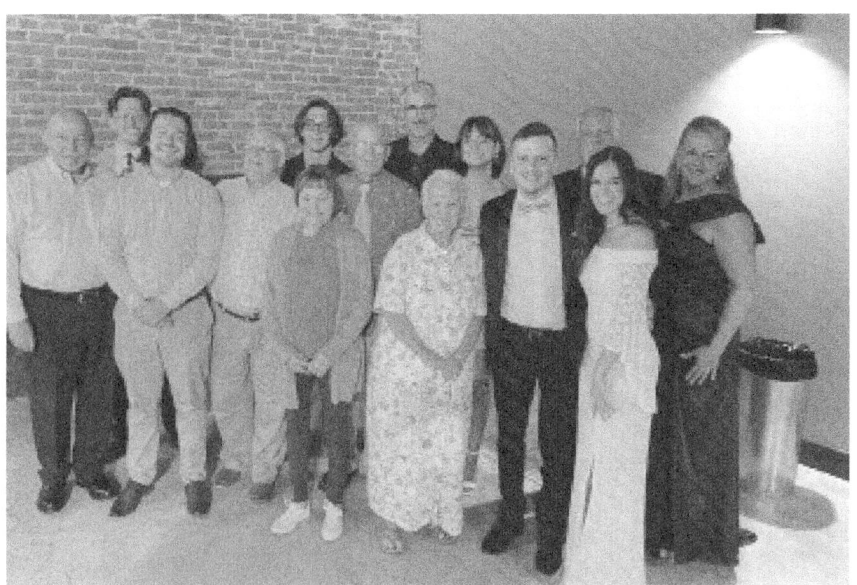

Martin family at the wedding celebration.

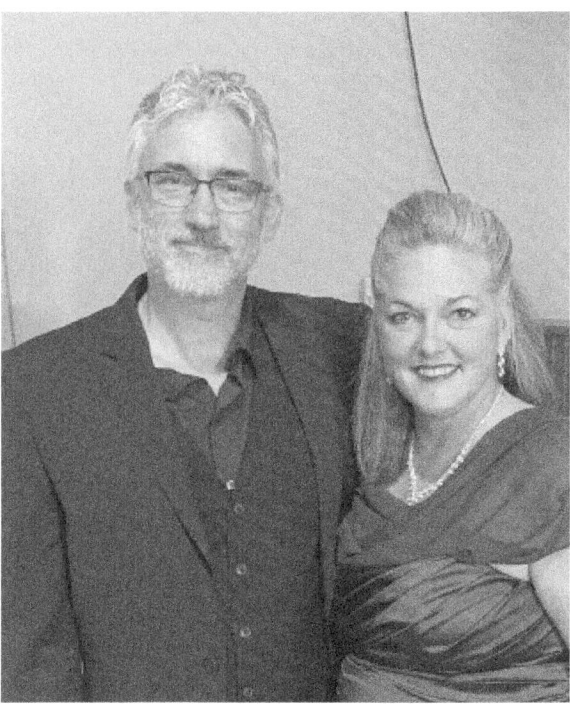

Cousin Tod McCoy and Brooke at the wedding celebration.

Our Love Multiplied

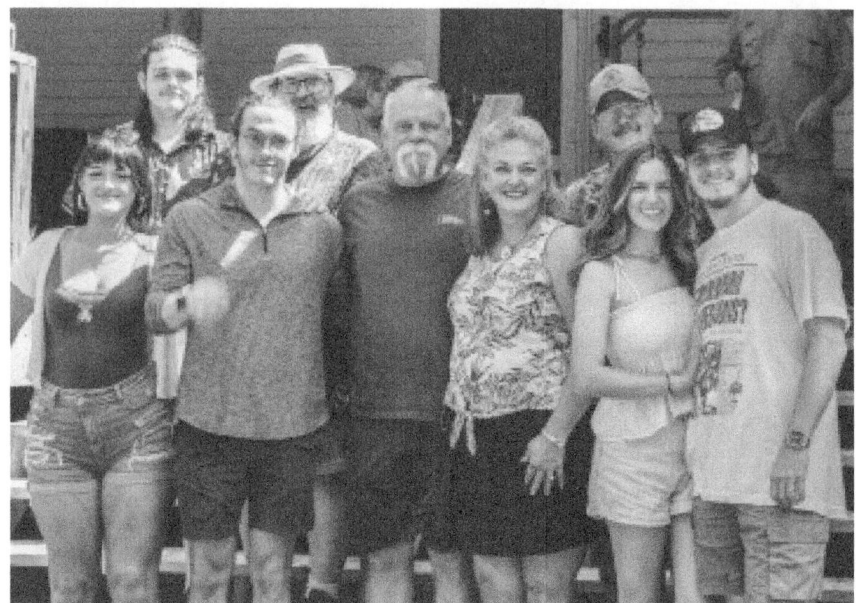

Everyone at the Martin family reunion. Back row (L-R) Peter, Trey, and Matthew. Front Row (L-R) Lauren, Thomas, Chris, Brooke, Nora, and Christopher.

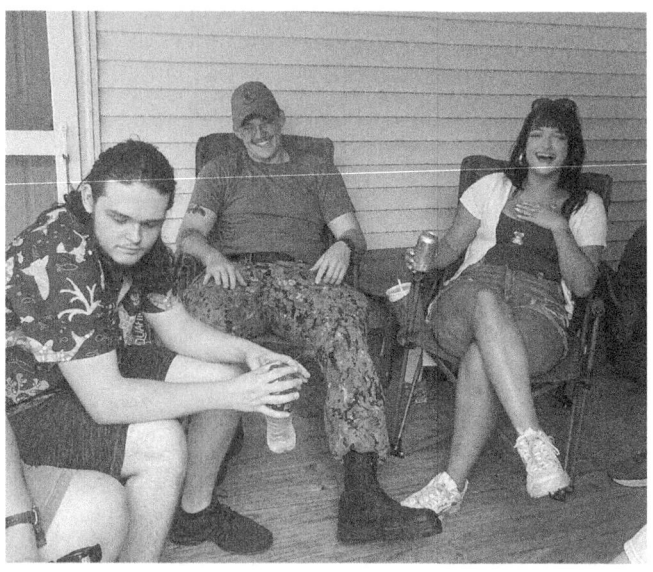

Cutting up at the Martin family reunion.
(L-R) Peter, Matthew and Lauren.

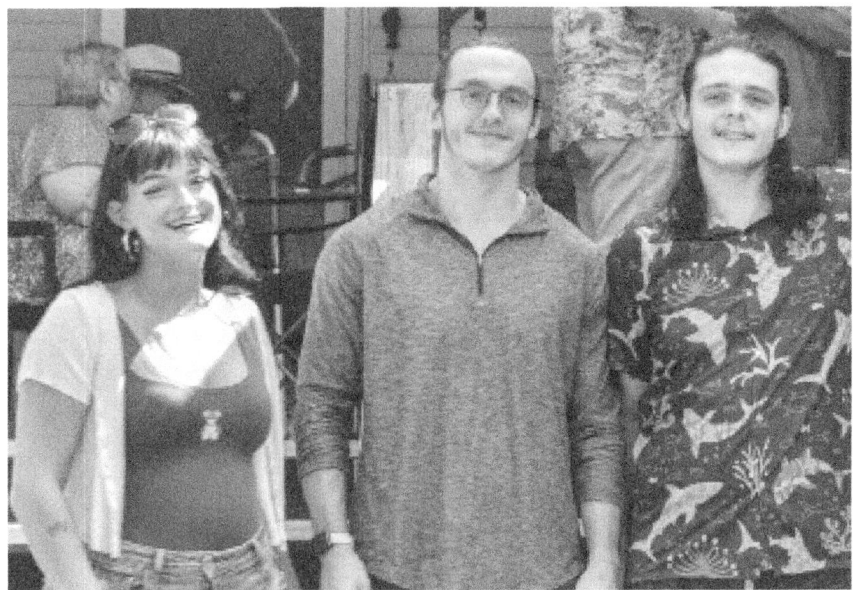

Lauren, Thomas, and Peter at the Martin family reunion

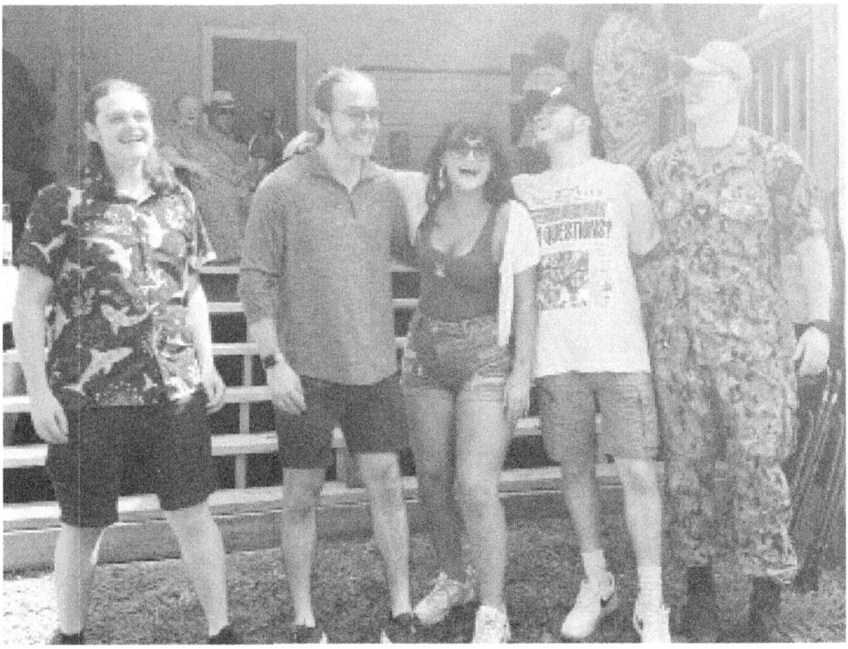

All of the siblings at the family reunion. (L-R) Peter, Thomas, Lauren, Christopher, and Matthew.

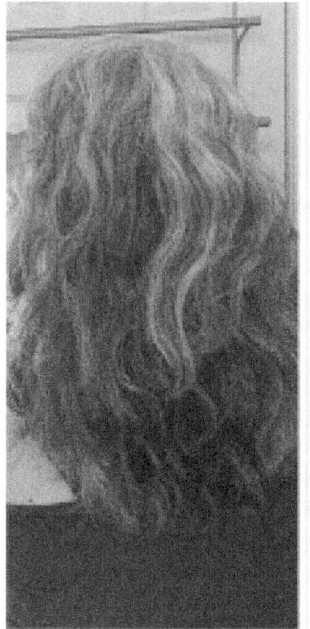 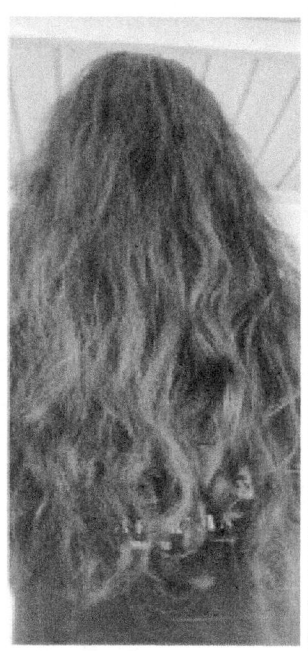

Strong hair genes: Brooke (L) and Peter (R).

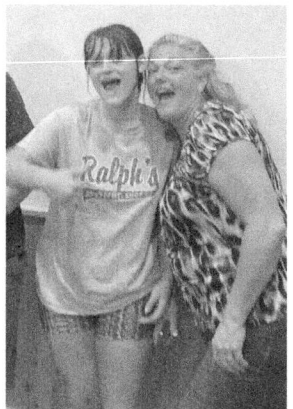

Lauren and Brooke.

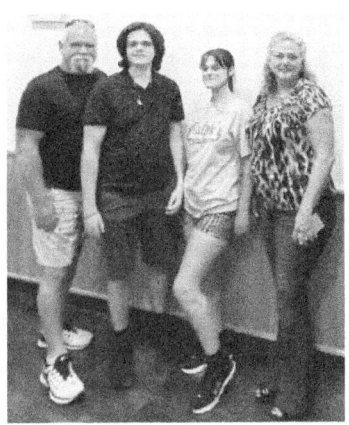

First time meeting Peter in
Nashville. (L-R) Chris, Peter,
Lauren, and Brooke.

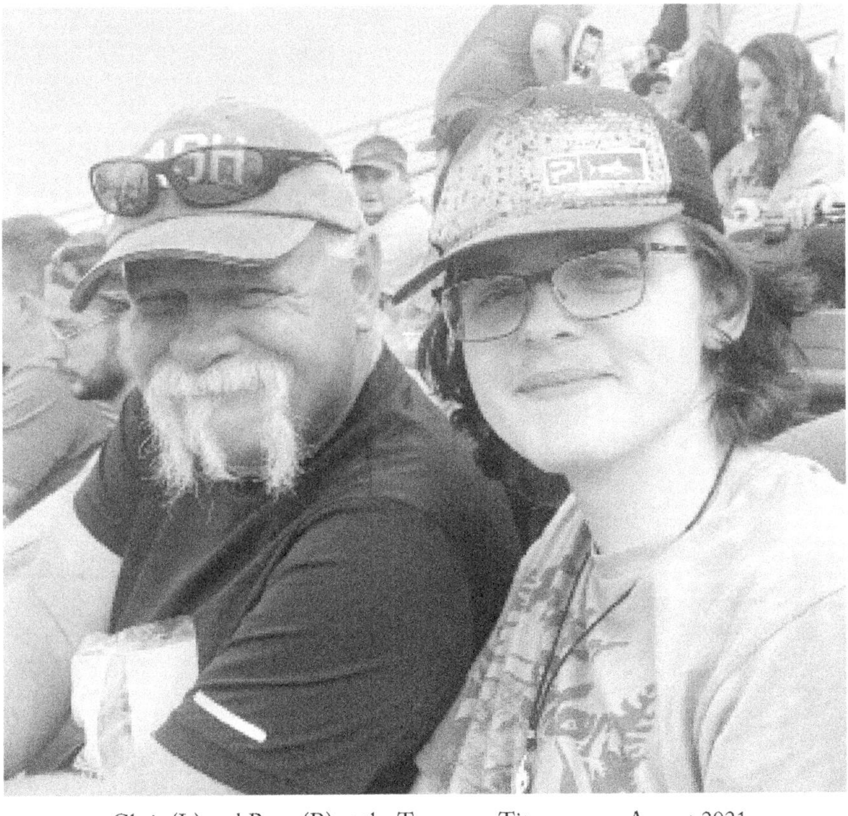

Chris (L) and Peter (R) at the Tennessee Titans game, August 2021.

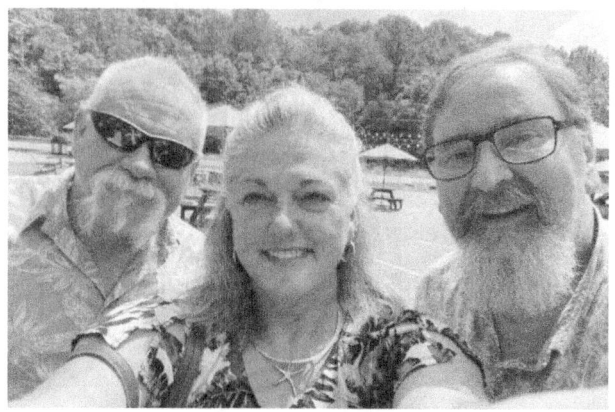

Brooke, Chris, and Trey's first meeting, Nashville, TN (2021).

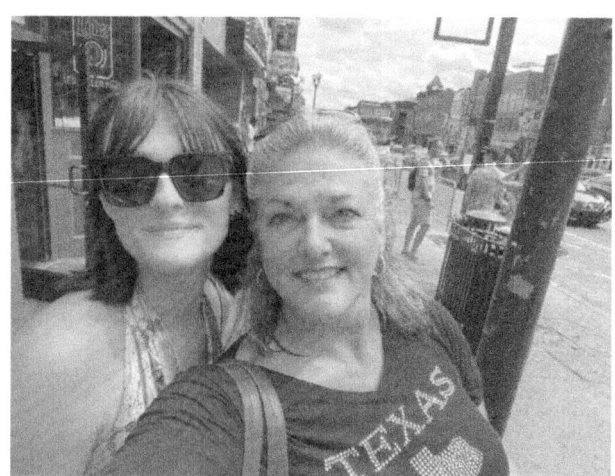

Lauren and Brooke in Nashville, October 2022.

Part 5—Full Circle

In October 2023, the passion to share our story grew stronger, and I started to write this book. I had experienced some writer's block, feeling that my words could never adequately give the glory to God that was due. I woke up every day with the urge to push forward, but I didn't know how. I had shared my story to a few small groups in Houston, but the deeper meaning was still coming together. There was something bigger that was stirring in my mind and my soul. It kept me awake at night.

My day job was keeping me very busy and was emotionally draining. I spent hours every day helping others finding mental health and substance abuse treatment. Public speaking was something I loved to do too, and I was a well-respected professional. But sharing this story was very raw. Very real. Trying to finish the book, in itself, had been an emotional journey with months of not writing. I wanted so badly to spread our story of joy, but I seemed to be frozen.

I have always been an assertive person—successful in sales positions and have never met a stranger. However, I have learned over a lifetime that many times I push when God doesn't want me to. So, I was just waiting on God to tell me "go!"

When Chris and I were attending Trinity Assembly church in Cookeville during the time we went through IVF, Pastor Jason Yarbrough and his wife Susan became our good friends. Since our story had become public, Chris and I had reconnected with them on social media. Over the years they had moved around the country and served at other churches. Eventually, God led them back to Cookeville, and they were now miraculously the lead pastors at the newly named Hope Church, former Trinity Assembly. In October 2023, I let Susan know that I would love to share the story again with the congregation. Later that week, Susan contacted me asking if I could come share my story on Mother's Day, 2024: Twenty-three years after I had spoken on Mother's Day, 2001.

And God said—"GO!"

I procrastinated preparing my presentation for that day. Was it a sermon? Was it a story? Was it a PowerPoint presentation? No, I thought, it was a message. A message for hopeful moms. But I couldn't quite figure out how to verbalize it.

One day in April 2024, I was at a local conference manning a vendor table involving my job and talking to a lot of different people. There was a young woman there who was also working at her vendor table, and I found out she had a six-month-old baby girl. She beamed when she talked about her baby and showed me pictures. But she also said she was tired, and I could tell that she was looking for encouragement and support. I told her that I had raised twin boys and I understood how tiring it can be, then told her a short version of my story. She looked at me with tears in her eyes and said that she hoped that she was being a good mom, and she hugged and thanked me.

The next thing I said to her came to me like God was whispering in my ear, and I knew that it would become my subject of my talk on Mother's Day.

"God created that child for you, and you are the perfect mom for her. You're perfectly equipped for her, and you can do this!"

That Mother's Day in Tennessee was surreal. Although Matthew was stationed in San Diego by then and could not come, and Christopher's schedule was too hectic to travel to Tennessee, we were joined in church by Trey, Peter, Lauren, and her boyfriend Daniel. We were also surrounded by many of Chris' family members from Sparta, including his sister Becky, brother Buck, and their spouses.

As I stood before that congregation, I talked about those days full of faith and hope 23 years ago when we were a part of the congregation there, sang in the choir, and received so much support on our infertility journey. Then I updated them on what God has been up to. As I explained the story, from my days at Trinity Assembly praying for my babies and those embryos, all the way up to the events to that day, I saw the joy in people's eyes and the amazement of what God has done. I showed pictures of my boys growing up—many of them had not seen them since they were two years old, when we had moved from Tennessee to Colorado. After telling how the story unfolded, I shared the comparison pictures between my boys and the Monroes on the big screen in the sanctuary.

I decided at the last minute to include the video of Christopher and Lauren singing together—that same one-minute video that I was sent less than a week after the discovery of the Monroes. It highlighted their incredible voices melding together. After showing the video, the congregation spontaneously erupted in applause. Jason, the former music pastor/now head pastor, was wide-eyed and later told me that it was the most incredible sibling harmony he had ever heard.

The message God had given me for that day resonated throughout my talk. The babies that God had chosen—for me. The babies that He had chosen for the Monroes. And the babies that might still be unknown to us. God had literally chosen each one for us, and as hard as motherhood was at times over the years for both families, they were given as a gift to complete a perfect puzzle that we couldn't have seen all those years ago. The unseen faith that we all had didn't have to be explained or validated. It was proven.

Part of my message that Sunday included the following:

"Moms: God chooses our children for us... and you for them. If you are struggling as a new mom, a mom of a toddler, a teenager, or even a grown child, know that God chose those babies for you. He therefore equipped you perfectly for the role as their mother. Mary questioned that God chose her to bear the savior at first, but God knew what he was doing. And Mary knew. She pondered and kept many things in her heart.

Not only that, but God has a plan for your children that is so much better than anything you can imagine, even in the hard times and tragedies we may go through with our kids, in our day-to-day struggle to sometimes survive parenting (believe me I have been there). God loves them even more than you do.

Think of that—and he knows YOU are the one that is perfect for them! What if the best thing you could imagine for your children wasn't even 10% as good as what God has in store for them?

My experience has forced my type-A, controlling, go-get-em personality to chill out and know every day that truly—God's got this! Moms—God's got this!"

On that Mother's Day, my heart was also bursting with gratitude toward Becky Monroe. As I showed her picture along with her triplets when they were babies, I looked over at the Monroes and saw pain in their eyes of missing Becky, but also a knowledge that this was all God's plan. At the end of my story, I had a special surprise for everyone. I invited Lauren, my daughter, to the stage to read from a journal that Becky had written in while she was pregnant.

Lauren read Becky's words:

"I usually avoid keeping a journal for many reasons, but I want to keep this journal to remind my children how I love them and want them all."

"We scheduled an ultrasound to see how the babies were doing. But instead, we were rushed to the ER because we thought we were losing them. We prayed so hard and asked God to save our babies. The ultrasound showed all three embryos doing fine—in fact they had heartbeats. That made everything seem real, finally."

Within that journal, there were quotes for the writer to read and reflect on. Lauren continued reading what Becky had written, saying *"This quote from Albert Einstein is so true."*

"How strange is the lot of us mortals! Each of us is here for a brief sojourn; for what purpose he knows not, though he senses it. But without deeper reflection one knows from daily life that one exists for other people." -Albert Einstein.

Becky's last entry in her journal summed up what everyone told me about her character:

"I feel as if I'm finally seeing my purpose in life. It's not to be rich or famous, but to be the best wife, mother and friend I can be to the people I love. And I do love you, my children."

As Lauren walked back to sit down to the sound of applause, I looked down at a beautiful scene: my newfound family sitting in the church where we had prayed so hard for life.

Our Love Multiplied

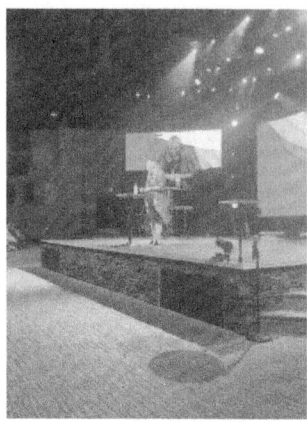

Brooke telling the story at Hope Church, former Trinity Assembly, in Algood, TN, May 2024.

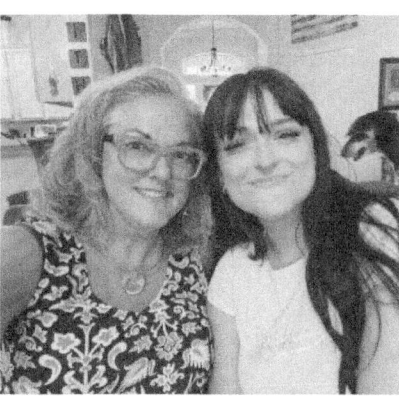

Brooke and Lauren, May 2025.

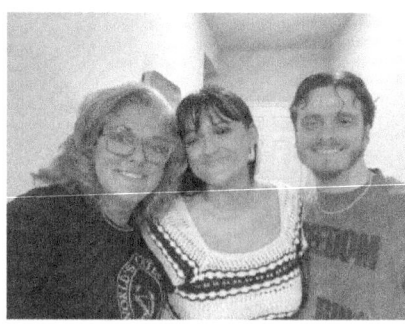

Brooke, Lauren, and Christopher. May 2025.

Brooke and Lauren, May 2025.

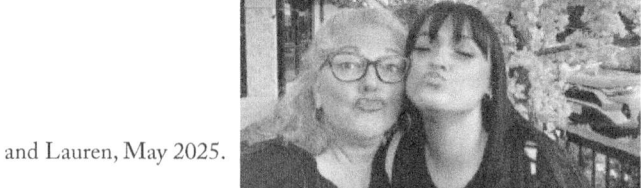

Epilogue

Whether you've never heard our story, or you have already heard it and want to know more, my hope is to leave you with feelings of joy, hope, and a belief in the sovereignty of an all-knowing God.

The purpose of this book is simple: to tell our story. It is a complete story in itself, with no room to create divisiveness or opinions regarding politics, religious beliefs, or otherwise. However, given the timing of the publication of this book, with so much in the news about embryos, I can't ignore the fact that many may think that I have a political or moral agenda.

Everyone creates their own belief system based on what they've experienced in their life or the lives of people that are close to them. Can you imagine if, after living my story, I would believe anything other than embryos are the beginning of life? My hope is that our story also makes you stop and ponder the same thing. Society can push opinions on us based on the current mood of the day. But deep in the human heart, at our core, we all know right from wrong and good from evil. I truly believe that.

About God's sovereignty: the word sovereignty means ultimate power. Throughout the Bible, God's sovereignty is referred to hundreds of times, and in the book of Ezekiel alone over 200 times. I believe God is all powerful and all-knowing outside of time and is responsible for the creation of everything. God has the power and knowledge to do whatever he wants or prevent anything he chooses to prevent. At the same time, the Bible says that God does offer us choices and holds us responsible for our decisions. God's permissive will allows us free choices, but yet throughout all of the bad choices we make, he chooses to bless us more than we could ever imagine.

There are many times I have wondered why God blessed me with this beautiful story. Although they're not all included in this book, there have been many bad choices in my life, lots of bounce backs from bad situations and stupid decisions, some resilience and sorrow, some shame and humility that God has helped turn to joy and redemption. People have told me that God's blessings are due to the choices that we made to donate the embryos, but many people have done that. All of the intricacies of God's blessings sometimes make no sense to me. It is because of God's grace and mercy, and that ALONE, that he has chosen to allow this blessing.

Isn't it interesting how we can look back on our lives and see how God has put things in the exact order that we needed? If things had happened out of order, we would not grow and mature as humans. But because he stacked our Jenga blocks in the exact way we needed, and even let them fall a few times before they were rebuilt, we can be stronger than we ever imagined and handle things that we never thought were possible.

When I was a young girl, my father was an orchestra conductor. I went to many grand concerts and even to ballets where I watched the orchestra and ballerinas move in unison. Sometimes, in the orchestra halls with the phonics bouncing off the walls, I would just close my eyes and let the music move through me. It was bigger than life, and I always wondered how the walls of the concert halls kept from falling down.

I envision God as being the conductor of an orchestra of lives, the baton in his hand, raising it up and hesitating in anticipation of the next move. He knows the next sounds; He wrote it all!

God's orchestra is carefully composed with many different instruments, all making their own unique sounds, blending and choreographed together, somehow in perfect harmony. Sometimes the music will crescendo and become exciting and active, at other times it will diminish until you can hear your own heart beating, waiting for the next note.

Concertos have different sections called movements. One may be completely separate from another but somehow mold together in perfect harmony. Just like our lives. There are so many different phases including growth, pain, joy, and sorrow. Just when we think we've learned it all, something else happens to move us to the next level of understanding. What a beautiful orchestra God has made and continues making every moment.

Thank you for taking the time to read our book. I ask that you tell others about it—not just about the story, but about the joy that inhabits it and the sovereignty of God that is evident throughout. I hope that it brings you peace, contentment, thankfulness and possibly a renewed faith that the complex orchestra of your life is still being played, and it is beautiful.

"Be still, and know that I am God: I will be exalted among the nations, I will be exalted in the earth." —Psalm 46:10

For more pictures, videos and updated information on the Martin and Monroe story, resources and support for embryo donation and adoption, and media contact information, visit www.ourlovemultiplied.org.

Made in the USA
Coppell, TX
21 February 2026

72024902R00090